BLW Baby Food Cookbook

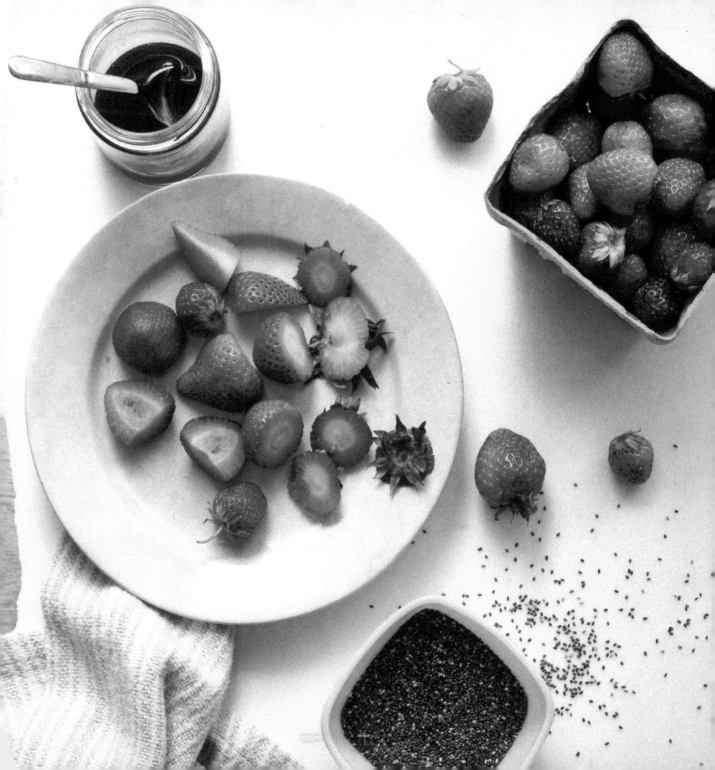

BLW BABY FOOD COOKBOOK

A STAGE-BY-STAGE APPROACH TO BABY-LED WEANING WITH CONFIDENCE

Ellen Gipson, MA, RDN, LD, and
Laura Morton, MS, RDN, LD

Photography by Tara Donne

ROCKRIDGE PRESS

For general information on our other products and services or to obtain technical support, please contact our Customer Care Department within the United States at (866) 744-2665, or outside the United States at (510) 253-0500.

Rockridge Press publishes its books in a variety of electronic and print formats. Some content that appears in print may not be available in electronic books, and vice versa.

TRADEMARKS: Rockridge Press and the Rockridge Press logo are trademarks or registered trademarks of Callisto Media Inc. and/or its affiliates, in the United States and other countries, and may not be used without written permission. All other trademarks are the property of their respective owners. Rockridge Press is not associated with any product or vendor mentioned in this book.

Interior and Cover Designer: Darren Samuel
Art Producer: Sue Smith
Editor: Clara Song Lee and Lauren Ladoceour
Production Manager: Holly Haydash
Production Editor: Claire Yee

Photography © 2019 Tara Donne. Food styling by Olivia Mack McCool.

Author Photos: © 2019 Dani Brown (Ellen Gibson); © 2019 Austin Wolf (Laura Morton).

ISBN: Print 978-1-64152-427-8
eBook 978-1-64152-428-5

To our adventurous eaters

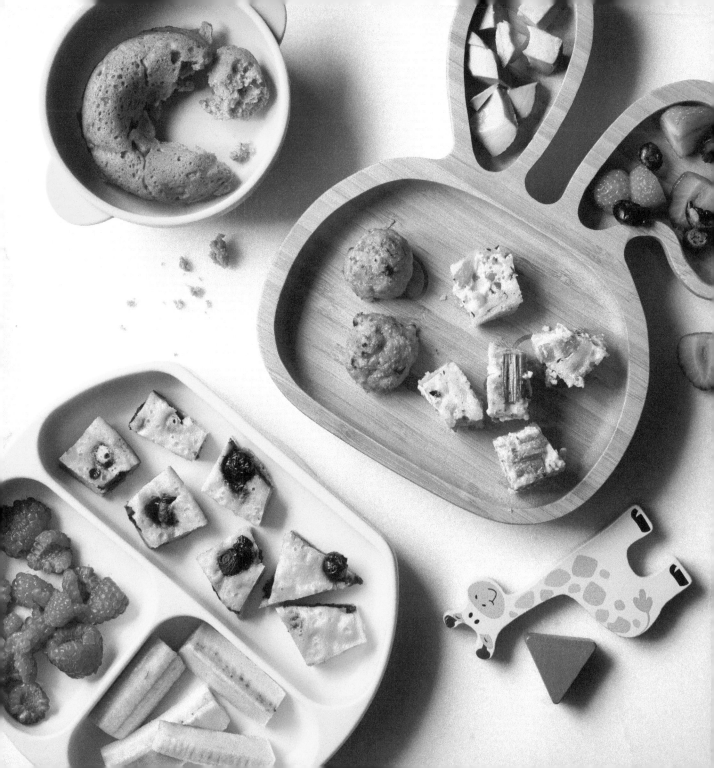

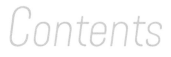

Contents

Introduction

Welcome, fellow parents and caregivers! We are Ellen and Laura, real-life friends, moms of adventurous eaters, and registered dietitians with a shout-it-from-the-rooftops love of baby-led weaning (BLW). Also known as baby-led feeding, BLW is a method of introducing solids that encourages self-feeding of appropriate table foods right from the start. It's a wonderful way of helping your little ones start a healthy relationship with food that feels intuitive and fun.

When we met, we weren't parents yet. We were both working as registered dietitians in schools where we witnessed a *lot* of picky eating. Children had trouble even identifying many fruits and veggies, and many had never tasted (and were afraid to try) simple foods like blueberries, avocado, or black beans.

We asked ourselves: *How can we help kids become more adventurous eaters?* It was a question that followed us into our personal lives when we became mothers. We concluded that the simplest strategy is early exposure. When infants are given the opportunity to explore, identify, and taste real, whole foods from the moment they begin weaning, they come to expect all these colors, textures, and flavors.

Ellen started her daughter's baby-led weaning with watermelon. A few days short of turning six months old, Ellen's daughter, Ruthie, abruptly stopped nursing mid-session to watch as her mother ate a slice of watermelon. Then, instinctively, Ruthie's chubby fingers grabbed for the fruit, refusing to give up until the sweet, juicy food was finally in hand. Ellen recalls, "I pinched off a tiny piece on my finger, and she pulled my hand straight to her mouth and swallowed, consuming a total of four tiny pieces. All of which were found in the exact same structure in her stools the following day. I could never eat while nursing again. All my food became her food."

Laura recalls her own child's early experience with food. "When the time came to introduce solids to my first baby, I watched excitedly as she grabbed a chunk of soft, roasted butternut squash from her tray and shoved it directly into her sweet little eyebrow. I was so unbelievably excited for her it never occurred to me to feel frightened or overwhelmed. These feelings didn't come until later, when I discovered websites full of BLW rules."

These examples illustrate the natural curiosity babies are born with and the importance of recognizing and fostering this exploratory spirit. But where should *you* start? You may have already started searching for baby-led weaning information online and found yourself drowning in pages of "rules," leaving you wondering if feeding a baby is way more complicated than you thought. Don't worry, it isn't!

It's common for parents to feel overwhelmed when it comes to the milestone of introducing solid foods. New parents can become so wrapped up in timelines, comparisons, and information overload that they forget to focus on the beautiful simplicity of experiencing baby's first foods alongside them.

Rather than worrying about strict, sometimes arbitrary rules, we encourage you to become familiar with this baby-led approach as a guide to developing a feeding tradition that fits in with your unique life. By simplifying the details, you can fearlessly help your little one establish a joyous relationship with food.

This book provides straightforward guidance on introducing solids drawn from research-based best practices and the experience we've gained by leading many families (including our own) through the process.

Even more, this book provides the resources to feel confident about setting your baby up for this wonderful and beneficial experience. It includes all the nutrition details you will need, along with our laid-back advice and insights and, of course, our most-used and beloved recipes.

As you read, remember that while we may be nutrition experts, no one is more of an expert on your baby than you. We hope you find this information empowering and allow it to supercharge your confidence in feeding.

Welcome to the table, baby!

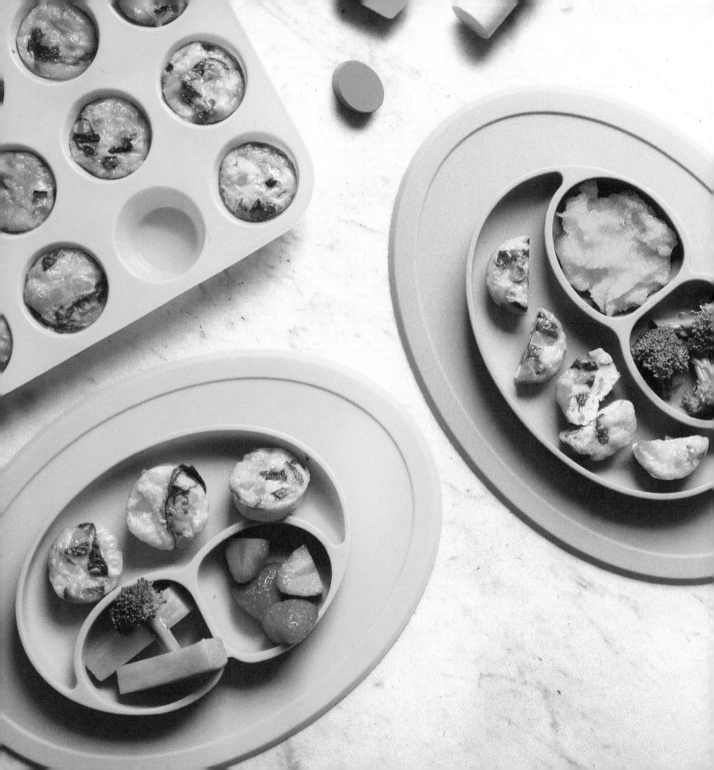

Part One

LET BABY TAKE THE LEAD

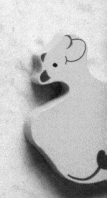

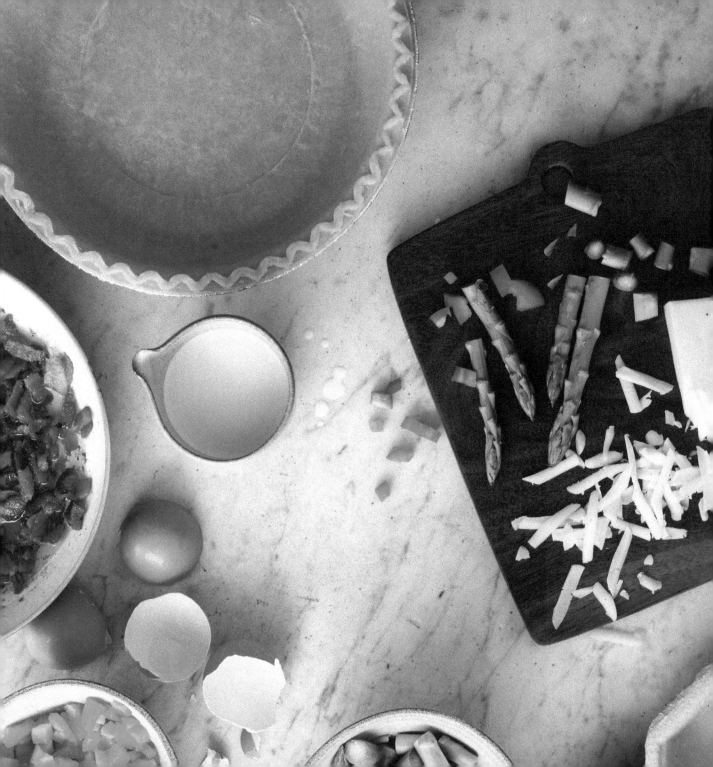

CHAPTER 1

BABY-LED WEANING 101

Starting solids can be a favorite milestone for parents as well as baby. Between deciding what food to serve next, shopping for cute new gear, and seeing your squishy baby "all grown up" in their high chair, emotions will abound.

This milestone is also special because it's the first step in a lifelong relationship with one of the greatest things on earth—food. Baby-led weaning allows baby to remain in control of their intake, setting them up to enjoy mealtimes. Parents and babes each have their own role in feeding. Parents provide the food and a place to eat, and the child decides how much they will eat, or even if they will eat at that time. It's helpful to keep this perspective in mind throughout the learning process, especially if you begin to feel overwhelmed.

WHY TRY BLW?

Although baby-led weaning may seem trendy, it has been used for centuries. Long before baby food commercials and parenting Facebook groups, moms around the world introduced solids by offering real food to their babies.

Over the past 50 years, the baby and toddler food industry has changed so much about how babies eat. Jars of food are labeled by stage. Toddlers are eating food labeled specifically as "toddler food." We like to think of BLW as a much welcomed back-to-basics approach to feeding. There are no special meals just for baby; instead, BLW offers a simple focus on nutrient-packed whole foods for the entire family.

Babies are born intuitive eaters. They respond to this intuition, which lets them know both when they are hungry and when they are full, and they instinctively eat the amount of food they need to grow into the body that is right for them. BLW is the perfect approach to preserve this incredible instinct and allow your babe to grow into a child with a healthy, happy relationship with food.

WHY BLW WORKS

With baby-led weaning, complementary foods are introduced closer to 6 months of age, rather than the typical age of solids introduction, which is around 4 months. Developmentally, this small variation in age makes a difference. Most babies do not need to begin with thin purées and progress through stages. Since they start a little older with BLW, most babies can head straight into feeding themselves soft solids at the family table.

We look at baby-led weaning as a guide rather than a strict set of rules. If you feel more comfortable including purées, you can do so in a way that fits in with the baby-led style. See the Purée? Okay! section (page 7) to learn more.

Talking About BLW

As a parent, you want to have confidence in your decisions, such as the choice to raise a self-feeding child. BLW is a practical, nutritionally sound, developmentally appropriate way to begin a lifelong positive relationship with food. Yet some may question you or even challenge your decision. So how should you best explain BLW to others, especially the naysayers?

Here is a quick baby-led weaning definition for family, friends, and caregivers: *Baby-led weaning is the introduction of nutritious whole foods when baby shows interest and signs of readiness to self-feed. This way, baby is included in the family meal.*

When you discuss feeding with your child's pediatrician, nutrient gaps may be their main concern. Share your plans to exclusively breast- or formula-feed until around 6 months, after which you will begin introducing nutritionally balanced foods for your baby to self-feed. Your physician may offer their own nutrition advice to consider, but, ultimately, the decision is yours. You may even ask if they have a registered dietitian on staff available for consultations to help address any additional concerns. They, too, may offer advice to consider, but, again, the decision is yours and yours alone.

When chatting with family, choking concerns and ensuring your baby is eating enough may be at the top of their list of worries. In this case, share the information provided in this book and assure them that babies around 6 months and beyond are developmentally capable of handling more than just purées, and they're also capable of meeting their nutrient needs by self-feeding.

BLW can also work for babies who attend childcare or daycare. Babies between 6 and 8 months old can eat breakfast and dinner with you at home and receive bottles at daycare before beginning finger foods alongside their peers.

BENEFITS OF BABY-LED WEANING

BLW is more than just cute sticks of avocado. The goal in baby-led weaning is to encourage the development of a lifelong healthy relationship with food. Other benefits include the following:

- **It may prevent picky eating.** With a focus on variety, your baby is exposed to many different flavors and textures that they can explore at their own pace without pressure. These factors are very helpful in building adventurous eaters.
- **It's practical.** No major prepping, steaming, puréeing, portioning, or storing is necessary. Also, no need to purchase any special foods. You can begin with what you have in your kitchen right now and provide meals that are typical to your unique family.
- **It is a great way to practice fine motor and oral motor skills.** Although babies progress without "practice" and on different timelines, handling foods of different sizes and textures helps develop hand-eye coordination, and chewing assists in developing facial muscles that are important for learning to talk.
- **It may lead to healthier eating for the whole family.** BLW puts the focus on whole, unprocessed foods with special emphasis on healthy fats and certain micronutrients. Because baby is eating with the family, it's common for the entire family to join in eating a more nutrient-packed diet.
- **It emphasizes the importance of family mealtimes.** Babies are born with the instinct to eat and learn, but they master these skills by watching us at the table. BLW encourages routine family mealtimes, which can have a major positive impact on the health and spirit of the whole family!
- **It builds an amazing relationship with food right from the beginning.** As dietitians, we often see mealtimes become a power struggle between parents and babies. A baby-led method means trusting your baby to eat as much as they need to grow, and consequently, establishing a relaxed relationship between parent and babe defuses this mealtime anxiety. When you allow your baby to remain

in charge of how much or even if they eat, you greatly increase the chances of a positive experience.

- **Encourages healthy body weight.** Allowing your baby to become familiar with and embrace their intuitive responses to hunger and fullness lets them grow into the body that is right for them.

Purée? Okay!

A baby-led approach to feeding is possible with foods of all textures, purées included. You can absolutely begin with a combination of purées and solids.

BLW is about fostering a healthy relationship with food while building self-feeding skills. The parent is in charge of offering food, and the baby remains in control of how much they eat.

If you're offering purées, try placing a preloaded utensil on the plate and encouraging your baby to handle it themselves (a feat that may happen right away but will more likely take a few weeks to master). It is also possible to spoon-feed while still carefully tuning in to your baby's responses, allowing them to remain in control of their food intake even though they're not physically controlling the spoon.

If you use a purée that comes in a pouch, squeeze the purée onto a tray, spoon, or self-feeding utensil instead of giving them the pouch to hold. This allows a baby to see, smell, and feel what they're eating.

IS MY BABY READY?

Every baby is different. Just because it's the eve of their 6-month birthday doesn't mean that they will wake up instantly ready and capable of self-feeding. Self-feeding should be treated just like all the other physical milestones. This is another physical skill that must be practiced and developed. No matter how much we coax, encourage, or bribe our babies to crawl, they're not going to do it until *they* are ready, and that's okay! Every baby is ready at different times.

The American Academy of Pediatrics recommends introducing finger foods once your baby can sit up and intentionally bring their hands or other objects to their mouth. Again, this is usually around 6 months of age. However, if your child was born prematurely, consider the original due date (instead of the actual birthdate) as the starting point from which physical milestones should be expected. But remember, all babies develop on their own timeline, so watch and let them lead.

As exciting as it may be to start self-feeding, getting started before baby is ready can be frustrating for parents and babies. Watch for the following signs of readiness your baby may begin to show when becoming ready to self-feed:

- **Sitting up independently.** This is when a child can sit in a high chair with good head and neck control and does not slip down if unsupported. This will reduce choking risk and allow them to swallow safely.
- **Absence of tongue thrust.** This protective reflex prevents the swallowing of unchewed food or other potentially harmful things like water bottle caps and small toys. This reflex naturally gradually diminishes around 6 months.
- **Increased hand control.** This includes the ability to see a toy nearby and intentionally pick it up (almost always followed by putting the item into their mouth).
- **Showing interest in food.** Your baby may show interest beyond just watching at meals by trying to grab food off your plate—no more can you peacefully enjoy a snack while nursing or offering a bottle! One day, a lightbulb will go off in their mind, and although they have no idea what it is that you're putting into your mouth, they know they want it. Get ready to foster and nurture this adventurous spirit for all of their childhood!

Never! So frequently we are asked if it's too late to start baby-led weaning. Maybe your child is 9 months old and happily eating puréed baby food, and you just heard about this feeding style. Perhaps your toddler is still consuming traditional baby foods at 14 months and presenting some feeding difficulties, so you're becoming concerned with picky eating. Either way, this book is for you, too.

You'll start with the same basics of self-feeding that we recommend at 6 months (see page 12). Let your baby smash, explore, and learn about food. It may take some time, and the transition might be slightly more difficult because habits and eating patterns have already been established. But they will eventually adjust. Generally, any time is a good time to create a healthy new norm for your baby and family!

NUTRITION AND BABY-LED WEANING

Making sure your baby is getting all the necessary nutrients is one part of baby-led weaning that can feel a bit overwhelming (even though we're dietitians, we have felt that way, too!). While the amount of information available on this topic can fill a book of its own, this book covers all the basics you'll need to know to understand just what your baby needs to enjoy healthy growth. We have also included a list of other baby-led weaning experts for you to reference (page 174).

For the first year, the majority of a baby's nutrient needs are still being met with breast milk or formula. Remembering this can remove some of the pressure parents feel when their baby is taking their time getting the hang of self-feeding. The term "weaning" indicates a process as a baby is transitioning from breast milk or formula to solid foods. Solids will begin to take on the role of primary calorie contributor around 1 year of age.

There are a handful of nutrients to keep in mind while starting solids. Including a wide variety of foods every day is a simple way to meet nutritional goals, but understanding which foods are good nutrient sources is important. The recipes in this book were designed with these key nutrients in mind.

NUTRIENT	PRIMARY BENEFIT	DAILY INTAKE (7 TO 12 MONTHS)	DAILY INTAKE (1 TO 3 YEARS)	GOOD SOURCES
Iron*	Brain development	11 mg	7 mg	Breast milk, iron-fortified formula, meat (especially beef and liver) and poultry, beans, lentils, wheat, oats, prunes, leafy greens, and blackstrap molasses
Zinc	Cell growth	3 mg	3 mg	Meat (especially beef) and poultry, oysters, yogurt, beans, nuts, and seeds
Fat**	Overall growth	50% of daily calories from fat	30 to 40% of daily calories from fat	Salmon, beef, avocado, nut butters, whole fat yogurt, butter, cheese, and oils
Omega-3s (especially DHA)	Brain, eye, and nervous system development	A few times a week	A few times a week	Breast milk (if the breast-feeding parent is getting enough omega-3s in their diet), salmon, skipjack tuna, sardines, herring, anchovies, or a fish oil
Vitamin D	Builds strong bones, plays a vital role in almost all systems of the body	At least 400 IU	At least 600 IU	Sunlight, fatty fish, cod liver oil, fish oil, and vitamin D-fortified whole milk
Water***	Hydrates the body, flushes waste products, and prevents constipation	A few sips with meals	3 to 4 cups	This is the only beverage recommended outside of breast milk or formula to children under 1 year old.
Salt and sugar	No nutritional benefit at this age	Less than 1g salt (400 mg sodium)	Less than 2 g salt (800 mg sodium)	Choosing whole foods over processed options as often as you can is a simple way to limit excess salt and sugar.

*Vitamin C-rich foods (fruits and vegetables) aid in iron absorption from plant sources.

**Babies have tiny tummies, so ensuring they are filling up on calorie-dense options is important.

***Be cautious when introducing other beverages (artificially or naturally sweetened) because taste preferences can quickly develop into expectations. Make sure water, formula, or breast milk are staples.

For breastfeeding parents, vitamin D drops are likely already a part of your daily routine (all infant formulas sold in the United States contain at least 400 IU of vitamin D per liter, so no supplementation is needed if the baby is formula-fed). Because of the lack of foods containing large amounts of vitamin D and recommendations to limit sun exposure, it is a good idea to keep supplementing at least 400 IU per day throughout childhood. This is especially important for those with dark complexions and for everyone during winter months.

FOOD REACTIONS

Every baby is adorably unique, and each will have their own perfectly perfect reaction to their first taste of food. Don't stress. Every reaction is normal, even the strange, silly, surprising ones! In the first few months, mealtimes are more about discovering and learning than actual eating. Self-feeding is a physical skill that babies must develop and learn with time. Sometimes their first meal can be anticlimactic, and your child may not even realize that food has been presented to them. Either way, have your camera ready for your baby's first feedings. There's nothing sweeter to look back on than a food-covered baby.

Here is a whimsical list of different eating personalities that we have come across in our practice. You'll soon know which one best fits your little eater:

- **The Foodie:** A precise eater who eats slowly and methodically and acts as if they've been having tea and biscuits with the Queen for years.
- **The Artist:** This child loves to feel and see food between their fingers. They'll likely spend the entire mealtime swirling, smearing, and sweeping food across the tray, creating a masterpiece.
- **The Destroyer:** Say goodbye to your beautifully sliced strips of food. They will soon be smashed and thrown onto the floor.

Solid Success

As your child nears the 6-month mark, revisit the signs of readiness and start planning for the big day they'll never remember, and one you'll never forget: their introduction to solids.

Here are a few simple strategies for successful mealtimes:

- **LET THEM JOIN THE TABLE.** A few weeks before you think your baby will be ready to start self-feeding, try to include them at the table to observe family mealtimes.

- **SHOW THEM THE YUMMY.** Exaggerate your eating skills and talk to your baby about the foods you're eating, how you're eating these foods, and why you enjoy it.

- **FEED BEFORE FEEDINGS.** Breast- or bottle-feed your baby 30 to 45 minutes before "mealtimes." Exploring with food is another awake-time developmental activity, just like tummy time, reading, and independent play. Likewise, you'll want to start with a well-rested, freshly changed, and recently fed baby for the best success.

- **SHARE YOUR FOOD.** Offer them the same foods as you are eating. Your child will want to eat what you have, so make sure you're eating nutritious foods that you want them to be eating. In short: Be the example you want them to see.

- **TAKE YOUR TIME.** Don't hurry your baby or distract them while they are handling food. Give them 15 or 20 minutes to explore. Your baby is learning about colors, textures, shapes, smells, and even object permanence; what might be going through their mind (and onto your floor!) are thoughts like, "What happens to this broccoli after I throw it?" Talk with your spouse, parents, and childcare provider about the importance of independence during mealtimes. It is so tempting to put foods into your baby's mouth for them, but it is strongly recommended that you do not. Children must be given the opportunity to try and even fail, which, in turn, gives them the opportunity to succeed.

- **BE RESPONSIVE.** Observe and engage with your child during mealtimes. Teach them coaching terms like "chew," "spit it out," and "swallow" to encourage safe eating. Watch for subtle signs of disinterest or fullness. These might include throwing food, rubbing eyes, and smearing or spreading food before the obvious cues of crying and tantrums.

- **COMMUNICATE.** Mealtimes are highly interactive and a wonderful time for introducing baby sign language! Between 6 and 9 months, many babies can start recognizing three to five signs, and by 9 to 12 months, some may begin signing themselves. Baby sign language is a great tool; it empowers infants to understand and communicate with adults long before their verbal skills develop. Our favorite first mealtime signs to learn are "more," "hungry," "eat," "all done," "chew," "water," "milk," "please," and "thank you." Babies may add their own flair and interpretation to these signs, and that's normal. They are learning to share and communicate their thoughts and feelings with you, and such a connection even before spoken words are exchanged is priceless!

- **The Social Butterfly:** First foods? What food? This little one is always intently watching everyone else in the room during mealtimes and may not notice that food has even been presented. This type of eater may need several "first-time" encounters with food before finally paying enough attention to get that first bite.
- **The Merry Maid:** A child more focused on limiting the amount of mess made than eating the meal. These little ones prefer self-feeding with utensils instead of their hands.
- **The Tank:** This adventurous eater can't be served fast enough and will (loudly) let you know it. So sit back, get second helpings ready, and let them lead. Just make sure your child swallows a bite before taking the next. You may have to start with smaller portions to avoid overfilling the mouth.

- **The Tortoise:** Oh, this baby is just quiet and content. This little eater takes time during mealtimes but will get the job done. Try not to rush; slow and steady will ensure they eat enough.
- **The Animal Lover:** In this nontraditional approach to self-feeding, these little ones have apparently learned by example from their furry older siblings. They see the food and just dig in—sometimes face and all, hands not necessary. Don't panic—you will teach them the right way to eat and proper manners, Remember mealtime modeling in the Solid Success section on page 12? Let them learn from you.

One of the best things about babies is that they have no preconceived ideas about how they are supposed to respond to a particular event—their reactions are uninhibited human nature. Whether they love or are terrified by something, their response is unique to their personality. However, as parents, we often have a whole list of "hows" and "whys" we think address what the baby is expressing. It may be simply because—well, your child *is* a baby. When it comes to introducing first foods to them, clear your mind of expectations and simply observe your baby eating food for the first time.

MEALTIME MYTHS

There are several mealtime myths associated with baby-led weaning. At some point, a family member or friend may offer their unsolicited mealtime advice, so let's prep you for it so you can offer an educated response, if even just to yourself:

"If they spit it out, they don't like it!"
Around 6 months, most babies will begin to lose their tongue thrust reflex (an innate response in which the tongue moves forward to prevent unwanted objects from being swallowed). Spitting may be caused by this reflex in action. Spitting out a food may also happen occasionally for older babies, especially when experiencing a new food.

"Ooh, look at that face! They don't like that food!"

Babies make all kinds of silly, expressive faces—they're babies, it's all they can do! Laugh, snap a photo or video, but keep on offering.

"You must wait 24 to 48 hours between each new food introduction."

Unless your family has a history of a specific food allergy, this "pacing" of foods is not necessary. We will later discuss introducing the top eight allergenic foods and the appropriate wait times for these (pages 18–19).

"You should offer vegetables before fruits."

One of the foundational principles of baby-led weaning is to introduce as many flavors and textures as possible. Preparing and presenting foods differently and serving them with different flavor combinations is the premise here. Yes, ultimately, they may prefer sweet, juicy blueberries over a savory mushroom, but continual variety and exposure to both are keys to long-term acceptance.

"Starting baby food early or adding cereal to a bottle will make a baby sleep through the night."

There is no research to support this statement. Throughout the day, it is normal for infants to consume small amounts of milk, stay awake for learning and exploration, and then sleep. Their digestive and nervous systems are quickly developing and need frequent feeding. Although many infants (bottle or breastfed) tend to cluster feed in the evenings, the frequency they wake during the night is related to the development of their nervous system, not the capacity of their stomach. The National Sleep Foundation states that for infants 5 to 6 months old, the main difference between those who wake frequently and those who sleep in long stretches was, in fact, related to the way they fell asleep. Learning to fall asleep independently (from an awake state) and having the ability to self-soothe at bedtime are both habits of infants with the most sleep success.

According to the Academy of Pediatrics, children between 6 months and 3 years old are at the highest risk for choking on food and non-food items. Children will put anything into their mouth—rocks, pet food, bugs, toys, paper, food from last week's lunch, coins, gum on the ground that is older than them, dirt, flowers, you name it—basically, anything they can pick up.

Emerging research shows that baby-led weaning does not increase the risk of choking. In 2016, the BLISS (Baby-Led Introduction to SolidS) study reported that baby-led weaning infants gagged more frequently at 6 months, but less frequently at 8 months, than did traditionally fed babies. This is a great example of the "Learn to chew then swallow versus learn to swallow then chew" feeding philosophy.

Gagging is a safety mechanism that closes the throat, moving unchewed food toward the front of the mouth so it can continue to be chewed. Babies have never swallowed anything other than liquid, so they must learn to chew their food and then swallow. Practice makes perfect. It's also important to note:

- Babies can also gag at the texture or flavor of a new food.
- Don't interfere with gagging by putting your fingers in your baby's mouth or quickly picking the baby up from their high chair. This can cause food to lodge in the throat or unnecessarily frighten them.

Common signs of gagging:

- Watering eyes
- Coughing
- Opening mouth with tongue pushing forward
- Sputtering
- Gagging sounds
- Vomiting

To be honest, a child vomiting is tougher on parents than on kids! Gagging does not normally faze babies; they will often keep eating, but when they do start gagging, remain calm, get down to their eye level, remove any other food from reach, and coach them to "chew," "spit out," or "swallow" the bite that they're eating.

Choking occurs when an object becomes stuck or hinders breathing in the throat, windpipe, pharynx, or trachea, causing a blockage of air.

Signs of choking:

- The child is unable to make sounds.
- The child begins to cough or their breathing becomes high-pitched and noisy—they may not be choking, but this may mean that something they swallowed didn't go down quite right. The parent should pay close attention to the situation.
- An older child (over 1 year of age) may hold their neck with both hands or panic.
- The child's lips and/or skin may turn blue.

Main safety measures:

- Avoid giving your child unsafe foods (whole, round foods, foods that break off easily, large portions of thick, sticky foods like peanut butter or cream cheese). Raw apples are the number-one choking hazard—whole or in wedges. See page 21 for more foods to avoid.
- Don't let a baby eat while reclined. This increases the risk, especially in rear-facing infant carseats.
- Don't let a baby eat while walking, running, or playing.
- Never put food in a baby's mouth.
- Minimize distractions during feeding.
- Make sure foods that can be bitten off in chunks when teeth arrive are half the width of a baby's airway—about half the width of an adult pinkie finger.
- Always be present while your child is eating.
- Take a CPR class to learn the proper procedures for clearing an obstructed airway.

All new parents are encouraged to become CPR-certified to ensure that they are mentally and physically prepared for worst-case scenarios; this certification is not just for their own child, but for the safety of all children they come in contact with. This is one of the greatest gifts you can afford yourself as a parent—to have this knowledge is the best insurance there is. Many hospitals offer free CPR training for new parents delivering there.

Digestive Challenges

As you have probably guessed, your baby's diapers will look a little different after you start introducing solids. A few changes you might come across over the first few days or weeks after beginning solids may include undigested fibrous foods or the skin of fruits or veggies, more formed stool with a stronger odor, way more poopy diapers than normal (especially when introducing fruits and veggies), and seeing a little bit of straining while pooping.

As babies adjust to the solid food life, constipation might happen from time to time. Symptoms include fussiness and spitting up more than usual, straining hard to poop, or going a few days between bowel movements. Here are some ideas to "get things going":

- Offer "P" fruits, like peaches, plums, and pears.
- Prunes (dried plums) contain a chemical compound called dihydroxyphenyl isatin, which has natural laxative properties. Try mixing prunes into a smoothie (see page 60) or chopping them fine and stirring into oats.
- Include a small amount of water with meals.
- Switch up the diet. Eating a wide variety of foods can prevent constipation.

Allergies, Intolerances, and Sensitivities

Babies and young children can be sensitive to certain foods and products. Results from a survey of United States households between 2015 and 2016 showed that the most prevalent allergens in children were peanuts (2.2%), milk (1.9%), shellfish (1.3%), and tree nuts (1.2%). The most common dietary allergens—known as the Big-8 allergens—are listed on the following page.

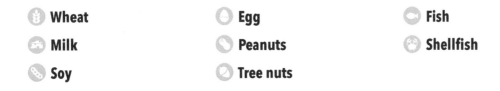

Wheat

Milk

Soy

Egg

Peanuts

Tree nuts

Fish

Shellfish

The prevalence of food allergies is increasing. In fact, over the last two decades, allergy diagnoses have risen by 50 percent. Introducing allergens is an important part of the baby-led weaning journey. Research shows that by including these foods early, you may actually prevent an allergy from developing. Delaying the introduction of allergenic foods does not protect against a food allergy and can increase the likelihood. According to the Academy of Pediatrics, the only research-based strategy in allergy prevention other than early allergen introduction is exclusive breastfeeding for at least the first 4 to 6 months of life. (For a great food allergy primer, visit the Food Allergy Research Initiative's website at FoodAllergy.org.)

Once your child has tolerated a few different foods, you can begin to offer foods from the list of potential allergens at any time. We recommend introducing these foods early and one at a time. For example, if you introduce peanut butter, wait a day or so to introduce shrimp. Once you know they are tolerated, offer allergens often (several times a week).

Peanuts are a great potential allergen to start with because preventing this typically severe allergy can be lifesaving. It is the most studied allergen to date, and research confirms the benefits of early introduction even for those at high risk of developing a peanut allergy. And if your baby has moderate to severe eczema and/or a confirmed egg allergy, talk to your pediatrician about peanut introduction, as they may suggest allergy testing or supervised introduction. (See pages 57 and 65 for good starter recipes that include peanuts.)

Rarely, babies can exhibit signs of allergies or intolerance after trying a new food. For clarity and safety, let's explore the differences.

An allergy is an abnormal immune response to a food protein. Symptoms can include hives, wheezing, swelling, eczema, recurring ear infections, vomiting, red cheeks, and sometimes gastrointestinal issues like gas, bloating, and diarrhea. This type of reaction is less common but more severe, making up about 5 percent of all allergies, intolerances, and sensitivities.

An intolerance or sensitivity is a more common abnormal response to a food or food additive that does not involve the immune system. Symptoms are often similar to a food allergy but less severe. They frequently include gastrointestinal issues like gas, bloating, and diarrhea.

Babies usually exhibit signs of an allergy within a few minutes to a couple of hours after eating a certain food. An intolerance or sensitivity may take longer to notice, sometimes resulting in an "aha" moment as you come to realize a pattern between a particular ingredient and tummy trouble or diarrhea.

If you notice a reaction when you introduce a food, hold off on offering that food again until you check in with your child's pediatrician. It can be helpful to keep a diary to share with your pediatrician in order to track intake and symptoms, especially if your baby is experiencing issues like bloating, gas, constipation, or diarrhea.

For babies under one year old, an elimination diet is the best way to confirm allergies, intolerances, or sensitivities. There is a test that can be done by an allergist to determine the presence of a specific type of allergy—immunoglobulin E (IgE) allergy—but it does not identify non-IgE allergies, intolerances, or sensitivities. But, before trying an elimination diet, make a plan to remove the problematic food for at least two weeks before reintroducing it, and discuss the situation with your pediatrician and/or a pediatric-registered dietitian.

According to the American Academy of Allergy, Asthma & Immunology, most children will outgrow allergies to milk, egg, soy, and wheat. The other four most common food allergies—peanut, tree nut, fish, and shellfish—are not as commonly outgrown. An allergist can help you determine if an allergy is still present by retesting IgE response and possibly reintroducing the allergenic food under medical supervision.

FOODS TO AVOID IN YEAR ONE

"Which foods *can't* I give my baby?" This is a common question asked by parents learning about BLW, but luckily, the list is pretty short.

HONEY: Honey can contain botulism spores that the gut is unable to handle until the baby is over a year old. Even honey used in baked goods and packaged foods (think honey-flavored cereals, graham crackers, granola bars, breads, etc.) may have been processed but not necessarily pasteurized, so it's best to skip these products until after age one.

COW'S MILK: Fluid calories should come from breast milk or formula rather than cow's milk, which has very low levels of absorbable iron. Cow's milk can be used in recipes, however, because it does not compete with breast milk or formula consumption. Other dairy products such as cheese and yogurt can be included from 6 months on. See page 129 for more on introducing cow's milk after 12 months.

CHOKING HAZARDS: There are a few general recommendations of foods to avoid until around age 3 or 4 depending on a child's self-feeding skills. Following mealtime safety precautions, including always being present while your baby eats, is the best way to limit the risk of choking (page 16). Here's a list of foods to avoid:

- Whole nuts, whole seeds, and popcorn.
- Large pieces of raw, hard fruits and vegetables, or whole small, round fruits or vegetables, such as cherries, cherry or grape tomatoes, grapes, carrots, celery, whole apples, or large apple slices. (Modify these by slicing thin, grating, or cooking until soft—avoid slicing firm foods into coin shapes.)
- Anything other than a thinly spread layer of thick, sticky foods like peanut butter or cream cheese.
- Whole hot dogs and other link-style sausages. (Serve fully cooked and cut longways.)
- Whole cheese sticks. (These can be peeled into thin strips or cut fine.)
- Whole raisins and dried fruit. (These can be chopped fine for children under age 1.)

How to Serve Baby's Favorite Foods

ACORN OR BUTTERNUT SQUASH–Halve, remove seeds, and roast until tender. Scoop out flesh, and mash or cut into strips.

APPLES–Slice thin and sauté, or peel and grate.

ASPARAGUS–Break off the bottom stem of thin spears, bake, and serve whole.

AVOCADO–Peel and cut into strips or large chunks.

BANANA–Serve whole, sliced into sticks, rolled in ground flaxseed or shredded coconut, or leave some of the peel on as a handle.

BEANS–Lightly mash.

BEEF–Cook until very tender and shred or slice into thin strips; or shape ground beef into patties/meatballs.

BERRIES–Blueberries and raspberries should be smooshed for easier pickup and halved for older babies. Serve large strawberries halved or quartered; smoosh or halve smaller ones or large berries that have been chewed down.

BREAD–Toast lightly, add a thin layer of high-energy fat–such as avocado, butter, or nut butters–and cut into strips or serve as a whole slice.

BROCCOLI OR CAULIFLOWER–Cook until tender, then cut into large florets with stems as handles.

BRUSSELS SPROUTS–Cook until tender and serve halved or quartered.

CARROTS–Cook until soft and serve in sticks or grated.

CHEESE–Serve shredded or melted atop scrambled eggs, pastas, grains, etc.

CHICKEN–Dark meat is more tender than white meat. Poach rather than boil, slow cook, rotisserie, or bake it in the oven. You can offer breast shredded or tender thighs or legs whole (remove all bones, skin, and cartilage).

EGG–Serve as a traditional scramble, as a scramble that has been cooked into a flat patty and sliced into strips, or boil and cut into thin strips, or boil and lightly mash.

EGGPLANT, YELLOW SQUASH, OR ZUCCHINI–Cook until tender and cut into strips.

FISH–Bake, grill (remove any char), or smoke until tender. Canned fish can be mixed into recipes or formed into patties. Canned fish with bones removed can be flaked and served on its own or mixed into recipes.

FRENCH TOAST, PANCAKES, OR WAFFLES–Slice into strips and dip into a yogurt and fresh fruit blend.

GREEN BEANS–Steam or sauté until tender.

MUSHROOMS–For small button mushrooms, serve sliced. For larger mushrooms like portobello, serve whole or cut into strips.

NUTS–Chop extremely fine and serve atop yogurts or in baked breads/muffins. Introduce whole or larger chopped nuts when you feel your baby is developmentally capable.

NUT BUTTERS–Spread a thin layer onto bread, stir into oatmeals or yogurts, or cook into sauces.

PEARS–Always serve very ripe, whole or sliced into thin strips.

POTATOES OR SWEET POTATOES–Bake whole and slice flesh into strips, or boil, or roast and lightly mash before serving.

TOMATOES–If using large ripe tomatoes, serve them whole or cut into strips; if cherry or grape tomatoes, serve quartered.

IT'S GONNA GET MESSY

One of the best things about this feeding method is seeing the pure joy on a baby's face when they play with food. As imagination develops, tomatoes can turn into lipstick, Greek yogurt might become moisturizing lotion, and half-eaten slices of bread may transform into wild horses. Their creativity is limitless.

For many first-time parents, this mess equals stress. But once you decide to just experience your little baby eating, exploring, and loving food, it all melts away.

In the first few months of food exploration, the amount that actually gets into a baby's mouth is very minimal (breast milk or formula remains the primary nutrition for the first year). You'll still want to focus on high-quality foods that pack a lot of nutrients in the tiniest bites because what little they do get in can go a long way.

Soon you will find food in every imaginable (and unimaginable) place: avocado eyes, crunchy yogurt hair, quinoa in the belly button, and maybe even a single corn kernel up a nostril. Babies are adorably mischievous little creatures. Here are a few mealtime tips to keep your kitchen clean(ish) and your mess anxiety in check:

SKIP THE WIPES. You could go broke using baby wipes for every mealtime cleanup. Save that money for a college fund. Instead, go buy a small package of soft washcloths in a bright, obviously-doesn't-match-your-kitchen-so-your-partner-doesn't-use-them-to-scrub-greasy-dishes color and designate them for baby cleanup *only*.

ACCESSORIZE FOR EASY CLEANUP. Some items that can become staples are plastic tablecloths on the floor under the high chair, bibs with a food-catching pocket, a cordless kitchen hand vacuum, a mini kitchen broom—even a dog!

BREAKFAST IN YOUR PJS. Wait to get your baby dressed for the day after breakfast so that a second outfit isn't needed before the morning ends.

STRATEGIZE BATH TIME. If your child is going to enjoy a particularly messy meal, it may be easier to serve dinner with them in just a diaper, then have bath time immediately afterward, instead of wiping food out of every baby crevice and laundering food-soaked outfits.

BLW ON THE GO

You are teaching your baby to become an independent, adventurous, confident eater, and that means giving them the space and tools to make each mealtime a success. Once they get started, they will not sit quietly in your lap and wait patiently for you to hand them their next spoonful of food—no matter where you are.

That said, we have created a "BLW on the Go Kit" for all your self-feeding mealtime equipment conveniently stored in one location. Keep this bag stocked and ready in your car at all times so you don't have to gather pieces on the fly while heading out the door.

Equipment Essentials

Basic drawstring bag—fill with:

- Small silicone plate
- Silicone bib with pocket
- Utensils (self-feeding spoons or toddler utensils, depending on age)
- Wet/dry bag (store plate, bib, and utensils in this bag)
- Small container for sanitation wipes
- Baby wipes
- Nonperishable snacks, such as dry cereals or crackers (depending on age)
- Toys, such as a small flip book, toy car, favorite teether, and drawing supplies
- Extra diaper and bodysuit
- Eating smock (great when you need an outfit to last past mealtime and for special events, formal functions, or going out to restaurants)

Use restaurant dining as an opportunity to eat foods you don't always have time to prepare at home. For instance, you can try seafoods like fish and shellfish; steaks; vegetables like pumpkin, eggplant, parsnips, beets, kimchi, okra, and kale; and other specialty sides. And, of course, be sure to first safely introduce allergens at home! Then continue to taste and build familiarity at restaurants.

TIPS FOR EATING OUT DURING BLW

Here are some of our favorite restaurant-savvy suggestions for building a balanced plate that your baby can handle. Try ordering the following:

- A side of fresh fruit, or bring some cut from home
- Steamed veggies with or without butter, or roasted veggies
- A side of avocado or guacamole
- Rolls or bread with butter
- A salad with lots of ingredients that can be deconstructed (like a Niçoise or Cobb salad, Southwest salad with beans, grilled veggie salad, taco salad, etc.) with dressing on the side
- Margherita or veggie pizza
- A deconstructable grilled veggie or chicken sandwich, wrap, burrito, or taco plate
- Grilled salmon
- White or brown rice
- Steak and mashed potatoes

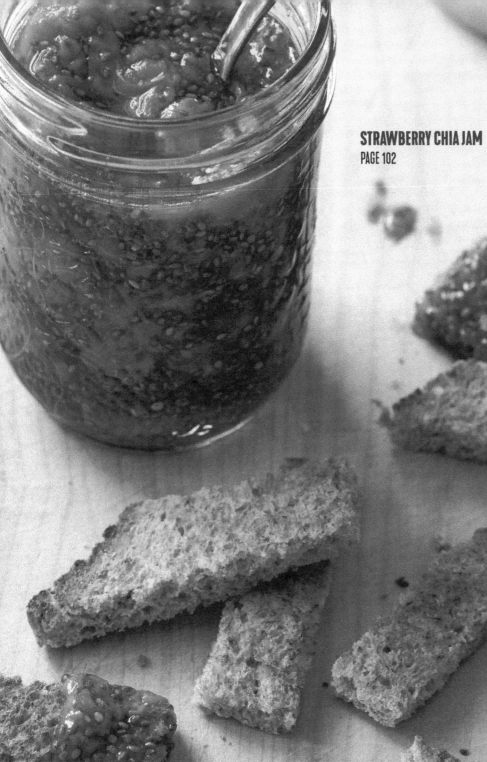

STRAWBERRY CHIA JAM
PAGE 102

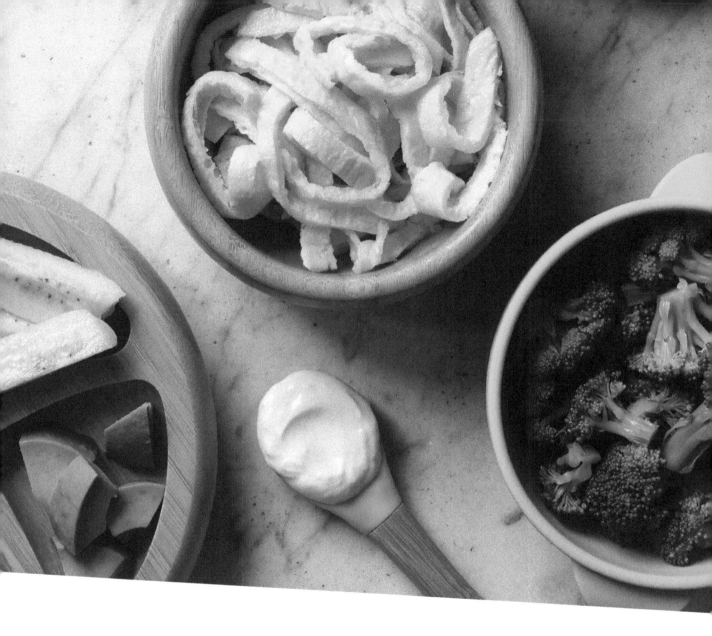

CHAPTER 2
PREPARING TO EAT WITH BABY

Now that we've chatted about some of the details, let's find the joy in what's about to happen.

While the anticipation of the first baby-led mealtime can be a really big deal for parents, the best thing you can do is set your expectations aside. Simply focus on being present with your baby and calmly offering support through mealtime. All babies tackle this milestone differently, and there is no one "normal" response.

A big part of BLW is the parental vibe during meals. Being as relaxed as possible and putting your trust in your baby's ability to regulate what they eat takes practice but is absolutely worth it—you're getting a front-row seat to cheer your child on in this once-in-a-lifetime opportunity, creating an adventurous eater, and building a "can-do" attitude at an early age.

WHOLE FOODS FOR THE WHOLE FAMILY

Because BLW focuses on serving one meal to the whole family, the quality of foods offered is important. Our definition of whole foods is simple: They are foods that are very close to how you would find them in nature. Not all processing is a bad thing; most foods go through some processing before making their way into our kitchens (like the milling of whole grains into bread or pasta or fermentation of milk into yogurt). For the purpose of this book, whole foods are minimally processed with a short ingredients list that haven't changed all that much since being plucked from the field, farm, ocean, or river. Choosing whole over processed foods is a simple way to get the most nutrients while limiting preservatives, trans fats, artificial flavor or colors, and excess salt and sugar.

Many families choose to go organic as well. Organic foods are grown or raised without most synthetic pesticides and fertilizers, growth hormones, irradiation, and genetic engineering (GMOs). In the United States, most organic foods are labeled with the USDA Organic or Certified Naturally Grown seal.

Whether you decide on organic, non-organic, or a combination is completely up to your family. In fact, even as nutrition pros, we have different preferences: One of us follows a mostly organic diet, while the other chooses mostly non-organic options. The most important thing is to offer your child a variety of nutrient-packed foods. Here are eight ways to get more variety in good-quality produce:

1. Check out your local farmers' market, which typically feature both organic and non-organic local options. In general, the shorter the time or distance your produce traveled, the more nutrients you'll find in it.
2. Look for "grown locally" signs at your grocery store.
3. Watch for sales on organic produce at your grocery store. Sale prices on organics can dip below the price of conventionally grown produce.
4. Seek out trusted local farmers in your community for produce, pastured eggs, and grass-fed meat and poultry.

Can Picky Eating Be Prevented?

As parents, we want the best for our children. But if we have a complicated relationship with food or are picky eaters, it's important to try to separate our own biases from our children's. If the parent already has a strained relationship with food, it can lead to the baby developing a negative relationship with food. A healthy relationship with food is where baby-led weaning starts. Babies have no preconceived notions, so the more flavors, colors, and textures they are exposed to, the more foods they will come to accept as a normal part of a yummy diet.

If you can relate, then BLW is a great opportunity to broaden your own culinary horizons along with your baby's. The concept of "one family, one meal" brings us together, makes life easier, and helps us all embrace and appreciate a variety of foods. We'll explore that next!

5. Search the Internet for community-supported agriculture (CSA) groups in your area. These programs deliver a weekly or monthly box of locally grown produce to your home at great prices. This is a great way to try new produce, too.
6. Consider trying out a meal kit delivery service. Preportioned, fresh ingredients make for super-quick dinners that can work perfectly for baby as well. Don't pay full price—look for introductory coupons.
7. Sign up for a produce delivery box, which contains produce that doesn't look perfect enough for the grocery store and is sold at a discount.
8. Try cultivating a spring, summer, or fall garden. Even just a pot of fresh herbs is awesome to have on hand.

10 FUN FOODS TO EXPLORE

Although the ultimate goal is diversity in your baby's diet, many parents prefer to keep first foods simple by starting out with single-ingredient options for the first week or two. Try out one of the ideas in the list below. All of them pass the "squish test"—they can be easily squished between your index finger and thumb, or easily spread when pressed between your lips. They also contain some key nutrients, including iron, zinc, and healthy fats. Use a crinkle cutter, if desired, to cut foods into sticks that are easier to grasp.

1. **Avocado**—Rich in healthy fat and naturally soft. Try rolling in ground flaxseed or baby cereal to make them easier to grip.

2. **Baked sweet potato**—Cool and cut into perfectly squishable strips.

3. **Ripe banana**—Here's a great trick: Peel the banana and press your index finger gently into the tip. It will naturally split into three equal sections; continue to follow the cut lines all the way down, then slice in half horizontally for a better shape for gripping. You can also roll strips of banana in baby cereal to make them easier to grasp and provide a bonus source of iron. Or leave on a portion of the peel to act as a handle (wash thoroughly first, and be careful to watch for whole, round bites).

4. **Ripe pears**—Peel and slice into thin spears. A ripe pear will feel soft around the neck.

5. **Plain whole milk yogurt (Greek or regular)**—Offer a preloaded spoon. You can also give your baby a scoop on a tray.

6. **Chicken**—A slow cooker is great for cooking super tender chicken. Dark meat is even richer in iron. Try shredding or even offering a leg with the skin removed.

7. **Broccoli**—Roast florets in olive oil, or steam until soft. Broccoli is an easy one to grasp by the stem.

8. **Roasted butternut squash**—Peel, slice into strips, and roast them with a little oil, or roast the squash whole and scoop out the soft interior.

9. **Tender strips of steak (cooked to 155°F)**—Beef is one of the richest sources of iron, so even if your child just sucks the juice out at first, this is a great starter food. Since oral skills are just beginning to develop, your baby won't really be able to take a full

"bite," but that's okay (see Steak, Really? below). Cut it into a nice, thin strip so baby can hold it with a palmar grasp.

10. **Scrambled eggs**—Make an omelet and slice it into strips, or serve up classic scrambled eggs. Use the whole egg for the best nutrition rather than separating the whites and yolk.

Some parents feel stuck on what foods to serve their babies after the early introduction period. We recommend simply moving on to foods that the rest of the family is eating, but modified to make them safe for baby-led weaning (see guidelines, page 22).

BLW

Steak, Really?

Starting at 6 months old, babies are only gumming and cannot take actual bites. Most are not working with any teeth, and that's okay! They get a lot of satisfaction from gumming and teething on harder foods, and it's great for developing jaw muscles. However, this stage doesn't last long, and eventually babies are able to bite a piece off and chew, so always watch them closely during mealtimes–they quickly progress in self-feeding skills and begin taking larger bites or putting (shoving) large or whole pieces of food into their mouths.

This usually happens between 7 to 8 months, making this a good time to transition to smaller pieces of food for pincer pickup (usually acquired around 8 months). As this skill develops, you can cut tougher foods into very small (diced) pieces. Your baby will be practicing picking up each piece individually (though some personalities will try a whole handful) and putting them into their mouth, chewing, then swallowing.

As always, avoid coin-shaped foods, and remember to make that sure foods are a soft, smooshable texture. See page 21 for foods that are not recommended at this age.

BUILDING A BALANCED BABY MEAL

The previous list of foods to explore (page 32) is a quick launch pad of ideas for introducing self-feeding of solids, and this time is more about introduction than sustenance. The majority of the food will end up being smashed, squished, or smeared instead of swallowed—after all, your baby has never done this before!

After a few weeks of bringing that banana to their mouth every time, and the avocado strips are no longer slipping out of their grasp, it's time to move on to new and better things. Thankfully, at 6 months, babies do not instantly require three meals a day. This is a natural progression, so you don't have to overwhelm yourself—just begin with one family mealtime a day. Breakfast, lunch, dinner—it doesn't matter, but if you can, make it a time when the whole family can sit down together.

BLW encourages babies to eat almost all foods, but that thought can be quite overwhelming when you're staring into the refrigerator. Where to even start? Luckily, babies don't know cultural mealtime norms and can eat any "style" of food, in any combination, at any time of the day, without regard for any preconceived notions. Talk about independent eating!

This freedom can make mealtime planning so simple. Think big food groups, small portions. Most infant feeding plates have three compartments, perfect for filling with a 1-2-3 method:

1. **Pick a protein/iron source**. These nutrients are very important for physical growth and brain development. Sources include cooked tender meats like chicken, beef, turkey, and pork; fish; eggs; or non-meat options like nut butters, cheese, yogurt, beans, or tofu. (See more iron sources in "Key Nutrients for Baby-Led Weaning," page 10.)

2. **Flavor with a fruit or vegetable**. Add color, texture, and nutritional diversity to a baby's plate with tender, ripe fruit or soft, steamed or roasted vegetables. Today's options are nearly endless, so get creative and try an unfamiliar fruit or vegetable each week. Make it a game—both of you can try out new flavors!

3. **Add extra energy.** Healthy fats found in olive oil, butter, avocado, nut butters, and dairy cheeses and yogurts pair nicely with quick-energy foods like whole-grain breads, pastas, and muffins, and cereal grains like oats, quinoa, rice, or barley.

Although it is a parent's wish that their children get a perfectly well-rounded and healthy diet every meal, every day, life happens. We all follow the five-second rule at home, eat out more than we'd care to admit, and sneak some candy before dinner. So don't put too much pressure on yourself. As parents, it is our job to offer nutritious, balanced meals to the best of our ability. But some days are tougher than others, and with BLW, it is the child's job to choose how much or which foods are eaten. Everyone has taste preferences, but consistently offering a variety of colors, flavors, and textures will cultivate a child's acceptance. Infants and children will all go through phases of loving a food to completely avoiding it for weeks or months, and then one day (as long as you keep preparing it), they'll gobble it right up. Every seemingly abnormal pattern, phase, or habit is normal! Continue offering a variety of colors, textures, and tastes, and they will become used to that as their norm.

Healthy Portion Sizes

Babies are born with an amazing ability to self-regulate their appetites by recognizing their own hunger and fullness cues. As often-distracted parents, we don't always get the message, so we can unintentionally train them to override their instincts as we continue to offer foods past their point of interest or enforce the "clean plate rule."

As you learn to tune in to a baby's cues, keep portion sizes small—1 to 2 tablespoons or the size of one to two adult thumbs of each food, and only offer two or three types of food at a time. Large portions and many choices can be overwhelming to some babies, especially new eaters. Allow second helpings (and thirds, fourths, etc.) if indicated. Let them lead during mealtimes, and watch intuitive eating in its truest and most natural state.

As you develop a routine and feeding relationship, you will become more comfortable with understanding what serving sizes work best for you and your baby.

Tasty Teethers

Just when you're getting the hang of this whole eating thing, a few new teeth show up and leave you with a baby who suddenly has little interest in food.

It's totally normal for babies to prefer breastfeeding or drinking from a bottle while teething, so don't sweat it if your child wants to sit out a few meals.

During this time, keep your baby at the table with you at mealtimes so they can continue to watch you eat. In the meantime, try out these solid-food options to help soothe sore gums.

- **WHOLE FOOD ICE POPS:** Pour a smoothie (recipe on page 59) or a pouch into an ice pop mold and freeze until firm.

- **STICKS OF CHILLED CUCUMBER:** Remove the peel once your baby has several teeth and is able to bite chunks.

- **FROZEN BANANA:** Push a popsicle stick or baby spoon into a halved banana and freeze until firm.

- **COLD, THIN STICKS OF RIPE HONEYDEW, CANTALOUPE, WATERMELON, OR OTHER SOFT MELON:** Here's a hack worth sharing. Cut a seedless watermelon in half horizontally, and place it flat-side down on a cutting board. Cut it across in slices ½- to 1-inch wide. Rotate the cutting board and cut lengthwise across the other slices. Repeat with the other watermelon half. Voilà, you've got watermelon sticks! Offer these to teething babies and the entire family. Keep the strips refrigerated, and serve them as needed.

If your baby doesn't seem interested in chewing, try offering soft, cold foods like applesauce, plain whole milk yogurt, smoothies, or whole fruit soft serve (page 63).

CREATING A FAMILY MEALTIME ROUTINE

Whether you're a first-time parent or adding a fourth member to the gang, a new baby changes everything. The importance of establishing family mealtime routines and the strong bond that it will create between your family members cannot be stressed enough. Mealtime is special—a time to share the day's experiences, tell stories, and make plans for the future. It's also a time to model healthy eating behaviors. Research shows that those who regularly sit down for a family meal have better language development and higher academic scores, are more likely to eat healthier foods and less likely to engage in disordered eating behaviors, have fewer depressive symptoms and less emotional stress, and are less likely to participate in high-risk behaviors. That is an amazingly motivating list! Inviting a new baby into the kitchen is the perfect opportunity to start your family traditions fresh. So turn off the TV, set your phones down on the counter, and focus on creating a healthy mealtime environment that you can be proud of sustaining for the long term.

Not sure where to start? Check out these successful family mealtime strategies:

- **One meal for the whole family.** This is one of the main focuses of baby-led weaning. No short-order cooks here—that is a slippery slope right into the pit of stress and individual expectations. Prepare one balanced and tasty meal for the family, and give everyone the right to choose or refuse what they will eat, but do yourself a giant favor and announce that alternatives are not an option.
- **Create a routine.** Children benefit from repetition. So, just like your child's bedtime routine, create a mealtime routine. For example, you might set the table and put the baby in the high chair while the rest of the family makes their plates and puts their phones out of sight; then put on the baby's bib, say a mealtime prayer if that's your tradition, and only *then* everyone eats. (This is just an example; set a routine that works for your family's specific needs.) A daily meal and snack routine also gives parents confidence to remind a toddler who asks for a snack 100 times a day, "We just had a snack; we will have lunch in 20 minutes," or, "We just ate breakfast, so snack time will be in one hour."

- **Delegate responsibility.** Letting your child get involved in the kitchen as soon as possible will do so much for their development and love of food. Around 6 months old, they can sit and play with non-breakable plates, cups, and soft, plastic self-feeding utensils during meal prep. Store these low and in convenient containers or baskets for baby's easy access. Once they start walking, you can ask them to go and collect their plate, bowl, or bib. Later, you can add in more specific elements like requesting a particular color plate or cup or asking them to help mix ingredients, rinse fruits or vegetables, and peel oranges or boiled eggs.
- **Establish expectations.** If possible, have everyone sit down at the table at the same time and get up from the table at the same time once everyone is done eating. They will learn that eating a meal is a process that takes time, but an enjoyable one nonetheless. When starting out at 6 months, 10 to 15 minutes is plenty for your baby's mealtime, but as they age, you might try to extend their time at the table to meet your family's usual mealtime. If your baby is finished eating before the rest of the family, clean them up and offer quiet toys like a book or coloring pad at or off the table. It may seem trivial at home, but that is where behavior is learned. Your future self will thank you when you eventually take your child to a restaurant.
- **Turn off distractions.** Make mealtime an experience your child associates with positive attention from you. Start by turning off all electronics. Get down to eye level with your baby and bond. Talk to your child about the foods they're eating, and ideally you're eating too! Even if it's not your real mealtime, sit down with those ingredients and model eating with them. Describe the colors, shapes, flavors, textures, smells, etc. And use positive reinforcement—say things like, "What a great job you're doing with those mashed potatoes!"
- **Try something new.** Set a goal to try a new food or different preparation method once a week. This can be fun for the whole family and keep mealtimes interesting! You may even encourage picky older siblings to sample something new if the baby is eating it.

- **Strategize.** As your child ages, you may choose to strategize and offer some of the most coveted foods toward the end of the meal so the less popular items can be explored and eaten first. You will learn your child's personality. There will always be foods your child prefers to eat—we call them easy foods. You can use these to encourage comfort at mealtime, or you can limit these during meals to promote exploratory eating.
- **Give thanks.** A thankful heart is one of the cornerstones for life and a strong parent-child relationship. Whether through prayer or simple acknowledgment, why not open your family's eyes to the blessings they are about to receive? You can begin your meals with thankfulness for whoever's hands prepared it, appreciation for the resources that allowed the food to be brought to the table, gratitude for a peaceful home to share meals with family and friends, and acknowledgment of the nourishment it will provide the body. Food is the fuel that keeps us alive, and every time a meal is made possible, we all have reason to be thankful!

PANTRY AND REFRIGERATOR ESSENTIALS

The following essentials can streamline the process of making baby food:

Refrigerated

Unsalted butter

Milk of choice (for cooking and baking)

Plain whole milk yogurt

Cheese (fresh cheeses like buffalo mozzarella and ricotta have lower sodium content than aged cheeses like Parmesan and Romano)

Eggs (all recipes in this book use large eggs)

Chicken, salmon, beef, and pork

Frozen

Vegetables like broccoli, peas, carrots, and greens

Berries, peaches, and mango (thaw or blend before serving)

Produce

Bananas (freeze some peeled chunks for smoothies)

Avocados

Leafy greens

Sweet potatoes

Potatoes

Carrots

Butternut and spaghetti squash

Apples and pears

Berries

Zucchini

Broccoli and cauliflower

Local/seasonal produce

Dry Goods

Unbleached all-purpose flour

Whole-wheat flour

Ground flaxseed

Chia seeds

Fortified baby oatmeal

Baking powder

Baking soda

Dry pasta

Quinoa

Old-fashioned oats

Chicken and vegetable broth, no sodium added

Canned or dried beans, such as black beans, chickpeas, pinto beans, and cannellini beans, no sodium added

Dried lentils

Pasta sauce, low-sodium

Chunk white skipjack tuna

Canned salmon without bones

Peanut, almond, or cashew butter

Canned tomatoes, no salt added

Full-fat coconut milk

Garlic

Ginger

Onion

Cumin

Basil

Thyme

Rosemary

Sage

Oregano

Parsley

Cinnamon

Any other spices your family uses

Extra-virgin olive oil

Unrefined coconut oil

Avocado oil

Flaxseed oil

COOKING TOOLS AND EQUIPMENT

The following equipment is useful for making the recipes in this book:

Preparation

Glass measuring cups (for liquids)

Stainless steel measuring cups (for dry ingredients)

Measuring spoons

Wooden spoons

Whisk

Silicone spatula

Sharp knife set

Box grater (for shredding cheese, hard fruits, and vegetables)

Nesting bowls (use stainless steel to prevent chips or breaks)

Food processor

Blender

Rolling pin

Silicone pastry mat or baking sheet

Set of small ice pop molds

Veggie crinkle cutter

Pie plate

Rimmed baking sheet

Mini muffin tin

Cast-iron skillets and Dutch oven (cast iron transfers dietary iron to whatever is cooked in it, especially when cooking acidic foods)

Deep 9-by-13-inch casserole dish

1 or 2 (8-by-8-inch or 9-by-9-inch) casserole dishes

Unbleached parchment paper

Storage

Glass jars and storage containers with tight-fitting lids for refrigerator and freezer storage

Reusable zip-top bags

FEEDING ESSENTIALS

High Chairs

After being around parents during this milestone for a few years, we've come up with a short list of things to consider when looking for a high chair:

- **Easy to clean.** Get a chair that has few cracks/crevices for food to get caught in—this is great, especially if you don't have a power washer handy!
- **Removable inserts.** If any part of the chair has cloth, machine washability is important.
- **Foot support.** Dangling feet can be a distraction during feeding and could cause your baby to pull a leg up into their seat for stability. If you have a chair that clamps to the table, you can position it over a bench or chair so your child has a place to set their feet.
- **Good height.** Keep in mind that your baby will be eating with the family, so a chair that is a similar height to the table is ideal.

- **Space.** Consider your kitchen size and the high chair's footprint. Some high chairs are quite compact and work great in small kitchens, while others can take up a lot of floor space. High chair seats that attach directly to the kitchen table are great for small kitchens and really keep the baby a part of the family meal.

Utensils

One of the greatest things about BLW is that you truly do not need much other than a high chair to get started. That said, there are tons of amazing tools out there made specifically for baby-led weaning. Here is a short list of some of our favorite utensils if you wish:

- **Self-feeding utensils.** These include the GOOtensil or ChooMee.
- **Baby spoon and fork.**
- **Silicone plates.** Look for a plate with three similarly sized compartments that lies flat on the table.
- **Suction bowls.** These stay put and are great for utensil practice.
- **Small, open cup.** An open cup promotes smaller sips and helps strengthen the same muscles used for speech. Learning to drink from an open cup (held by an adult at first) also makes it easier to transition to a cup with a straw (compared to a spouted sippy cup).

Keeping Clean

A few simple items will come in handy:

- **Warm washcloth.** Be ready to catch spills as they happen.
- **Pocketed bibs and long-sleeve smocks.** Pocketed bibs keep food out of babe's lap and off of the floor, and long-sleeve smocks keep arms clean.
- **Drop cloth or reusable plastic tablecloth.** Place this under the high chair, and then shake it outside or into the trash can after meals.

You may want to purchase some basic tiny food storage containers and use them only for the baby's food. Appropriate portion sizes are often much smaller than you realize, so a single peach slice, six green beans, or a few pieces of macaroni are absolutely enough to save and store for a quick lunch. Use this hack to avoid filling up the fridge with bulky, mostly empty containers.

Before storing leftovers, prep the food so it's safe for the baby to eat, such as quartering grapes or taking the skin off cooked chicken. Then it's ready to go with no prep or mealtime stress.

ABOUT THE RECIPES

The recipes in this book are simple to prepare and offer a variety of ways to introduce the allergens discussed in chapter 1.

Recipes may contain one or more of the following labels:

Freezer-friendly—Can be made ahead of time and stored for up to a few months in the freezer.

Dairy-free—Contains no milk, cheese, yogurt, or other dairy products.

Gluten-free—Contains no gluten, a protein substance primarily found in cereal grains and wheat flour.

Nut-free—Contains no peanuts or tree nuts.

Vegetarian—Contains no meat.

Vegan—Contains no animal products.

ALLERGEN KEY

Recipes also have the following icons to indicate the presence of Big-8 allergens. Look for these icons if you want to introduce your baby to certain allergens or avoid them:

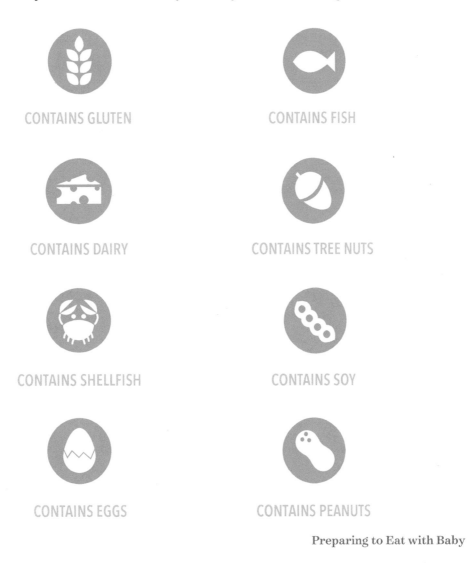

CONTAINS GLUTEN

CONTAINS FISH

CONTAINS DAIRY

CONTAINS TREE NUTS

CONTAINS SHELLFISH

CONTAINS SOY

CONTAINS EGGS

CONTAINS PEANUTS

BLUEBERRY LEMON
SKILLET CAKE
PAGE 101

Part Two

RECIPES FOR BABY

(AND THE WHOLE FAMILY)

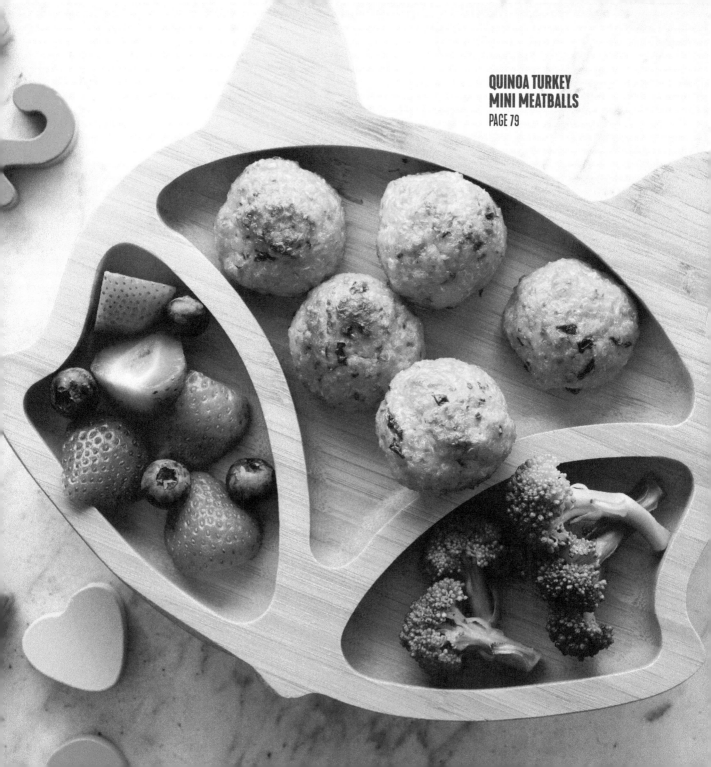

QUINOA TURKEY MINI MEATBALLS
PAGE 79

CHAPTER 3
6 TO 8 MONTHS
FIRST FOODS

WHAT TO EXPECT

We've discussed how, in the first few weeks of practicing baby-led weaning, little to no food may actually be consumed. This food will end up somewhere—actually, everywhere—so gear them up or strip them down and let 'em explore!

Some babies catch on to self-feeding quickly, while others need a few extra days (or weeks). Both are normal. Self-feeding, picking up items, bringing them to the mouth, chewing, and swallowing are developmental skills just like sitting up, crawling, or walking—each child will master them at different times. Progress is not dictated by birthdate, especially with preemies. Even if they are able to get some food in, babies might still be doing a lot of playing with food, consuming only a few tablespoons at meals.

The best you can do as a parent is provide adequate learning opportunities (in this case, mealtimes) where self-feeding can be practiced and your child's confidence can grow.

Baby's Motor Skills

Fine motor skills used for eating are quite limited at this stage, but infants will soon begin using their palmar grasp (whole hand) to pick up and bring food to their mouth or at least the general area. Safe self-feeding relies on good head and neck control and strong spinal posture when seated in a high chair. During this time, they may also begin the raking grasp, bending and flexing the fingers to move food toward them.

Eating at This Stage

During this exploratory phase, a lot of questions might come up. Remember that you are the expert with your child—don't be afraid to use that intuition, along with your baby's input, to help guide you.

The first question might be: How much food should I offer? A good sample schedule to start off with might include one or two meals per day at 6 months, moving along to two meals per day from 7 to 8 months. In the beginning phase, you'll want to start with a small amount of two or three foods per meal; for example, you can serve one slice of avocado, one strip of tender meat, and one slice of ripe kiwi. Play around with this concept and see what works best for you and your baby.

Give your baby a good chunk of time to explore—10 to 15 minutes is a good place to start. Rely on their cues to let you know when they are finished eating. If mealtime turns into throwing food or smearing it around without stopping to taste any of it, it may be wind-down time.

At this point, you'll still continue breast or formula feeding as you were prior to beginning solids. A baby's intake of breast milk or formula will not decrease much in these first few months.

Recipes at This Stage

As you begin to flip through the recipes in this book, you may think that they don't exactly remind you of baby food. We love that! We did it intentionally, because one of the most amazing objectives of baby-led weaning is one family, one meal. We want this cookbook to be a lifelong resource to you—past the yogurt-covered baby cheeks, the preschool playdates, the middle-school sleepover snacks, and the bottomless pit that is your teenager's stomach. These are real, good recipes for real life. We hope this cookbook contains what will become your family's all-time favorite recipes—because they're our families' favorites, too! Keep in mind that some of these recipes were created with limited added sugar and salt. Many families find that taste buds adjust over time; however, adults can always add these ingredients at the table.

If the thought of cooking from scratch seven days a week is intimidating, don't worry; we're not asking you to. (See our list of tips for eating out and on the go on page 26.) We absolutely want you to get comfortable in the kitchen but start small. If home cooking is not a norm for you, focus on a few home mealtimes a week and build from there. A lot of our recipes leave room for leftovers; take advantage of that option to cook once and serve twice or more.

The recipes in this section are perfect for beginner babies (and parents) because they are simple to prepare and pass the "squish test"—all recipes yield items that can be easily squished between the thumb and forefinger, making them safe options for little gums. These recipes also include introduction ideas for the Big-8 allergens that we discussed on pages 18–19. Along with these recipes, here are some things you can do to set your baby up for eating success:

SPICE AS USUAL. Feel free to spice food in the same ways you typically would, except for salt and super spicy seasonings like cayenne pepper. Using a variety of the milder herbs and seasonings helps increase babies' exposure to different flavors.

PASS THE SQUISH TEST. Make sure all foods in this beginning stage smoosh easily between your thumb and pointer finger.

PRESENT FOODS THEY CAN MANAGE. Serve finger-length strips of appropriately textured foods that can be picked up with the fist and still leave a little sticking out the top. You can also serve soft foods like muffins or fritters whole. Babies become pretty efficient with their palmar grasp and can get softer foods in that way, or you can offer on a preloaded spoon or utensil.

The recipes at this stage focus on the nutrients we discussed earlier (see the chart on page 10) and cover all the bases on allergen introduction. You can stick to combining single-ingredient foods (like those on the list on page 32) as you begin to include combined foods, or you can try these recipes right from the start.

Let's get cooking!

MAKE-AHEAD MINI EGG MUFFINS

FREEZER-FRIENDLY, GLUTEN-FREE, NUT-FREE, VEGETARIAN
YIELDS 24 MINI MUFFINS

Having these muffins on hand for busy mornings is reason to wake up excited for breakfast. They are incredibly versatile, too, so sub your favorite veggie, meat, and cheese combinations. These can also be made in regular-size muffin tins—just increase cook time to 20 minutes.

Butter or oil, for greasing

2 tablespoons extra-virgin olive oil

1 bell pepper, diced

½ onion, diced

1 cup fresh spinach, chopped

10 eggs

1 cup shredded cheese

1. Preheat the oven to 350°F. Lightly grease a mini muffin tin with butter or oil.

2. In a skillet over medium heat, heat the olive oil. Add the pepper and onion, and sauté until the onion is translucent. Add the spinach and cook, stirring frequently, for a minute longer.

3. Scoop about 1 tablespoon of mixture into each muffin cup.

4. In a medium bowl, whisk the eggs, stir in the shredded cheese, and pour the mixture over the vegetable mixture in the muffin tin.

5. Bake the muffins for 10 minutes, until set in the center.

6. Store muffins in a sealed container in the refrigerator for 2 to 3 days. Freeze in a freezer-safe container for up to 3 months.

TIP: This recipe lends itself well to variations. Try combos like black bean, Cheddar, and chopped bell pepper; goat cheese, asparagus, and fresh herbs; diced cooked sweet potato with diced fresh broccoli; or shredded mozzarella, diced tomato, and fresh basil.

EGG AND SPINACH OMELET

GLUTEN-FREE, NUT-FREE, VEGETARIAN
YIELDS 4 TO 6 STRIPS

This simple egg dish is an inexpensive protein- and iron-rich source great for any time of day. Enhance baby's iron absorption with a quick side of vitamin C, like orange or tomato slices, and cook it in a cast-iron skillet if you can.

1 teaspoon butter	5 or 6 fresh spinach leaves	1 egg

1. In a small cast-iron skillet over medium heat, melt the butter.

2. Rinse the spinach and remove the stems. Chiffonade the spinach by first stacking the leaves on top of each other. Tightly roll the leaves into a cylinder shape. Secure the cylinder with your non-dominant hand, and, using a sharp knife, carefully make cuts ⅛-inch apart, creating strips.

3. In a small bowl, beat the egg. Add the spinach, and mix into the egg to coat.

4. Gently pour the egg-spinach mixture into the pan, swirling to cover evenly.

5. Cook for 2 to 3 minutes, then flip and cook for one more minute until completely set and slightly brown. Transfer the omelet to a plate and allow it to cool slightly.

6. Slice the omelet into strips to serve.

7. Store leftovers in a sealed container in the refrigerator for up to 3 days. Freeze leftovers in a zip-top bag for up to 3 months.

TIP: Substitute spinach with other veggies you have on hand—such as diced tomatoes, diced broccoli florets, diced bell peppers, mushrooms—or just serve the omelet plain.

FLUFFY QUINOA PANCAKES

FREEZER-FRIENDLY, NUT-FREE, VEGETARIAN
YIELDS ABOUT 12 SMALL PANCAKES

This recipe was thought up with one goal: to make a pancake that won't leave you hungry again 30 minutes after eating. Thanks to the quinoa and oats, these pancakes offer a healthy and satisfying dose of protein. They are also very soft and fluffy, making them a great choice for babies from 6 months on. You can use any type of milk for this recipe.

1 cup cooked and cooled quinoa

1 cup old-fashioned oats

1 cup milk of choice

2 eggs

4 pitted dates or 2 tablespoons brown sugar

2 teaspoons vanilla extract

½ teaspoon baking soda

3 tablespoons coconut oil, divided

Pinch salt

1. Combine the quinoa, oats, milk, eggs, dates, vanilla, and baking soda in a food processor or high-powered blender, and blend until smooth.

2. In a skillet over medium heat, heat 1 tablespoon of coconut oil. Once hot, pour ¼ cup batter into pan. Cook until bubbles form, and then flip, cooking for about a minute longer.

3. Repeat with remaining batter, adding the remaining coconut oil to the pan as needed.

4. Store leftovers in a sealed container in the refrigerator. To freeze, place in a zip-top bag with parchment paper between each pancake.

TIP: 1 cup uncooked quinoa yields 3 cups of cooked quinoa.

PUMPKIN PIE FOR BREAKFAST

GLUTEN-FREE, NUT-FREE, VEGETARIAN
YIELDS 1 (9-INCH) PIE

We are always looking for ways to eat more veggies, especially early in the day. With this simple pumpkin pie recipe, you not only get to have pie for breakfast, but you also get a serving of veggies packed with a good amount of protein, tons of vitamin A, and even a dose of iron.

Butter, for greasing

1 (15-ounce) can pure pumpkin (not pumpkin pie filling)

3 eggs

1 teaspoon pumpkin pie spice

¼ cup milk

1. Preheat the oven to 350°F, and use butter to grease a 9-inch pie pan.

2. In a large bowl, whisk together all ingredients until smooth.

3. Pour the mixture into the prepared pan and bake for 20 to 25 minutes, until set in the center. Serve warm.

4. Refrigerate leftovers in a container with a tightly fitting lid for up to 3 days.

TIP: To sweeten this recipe, add in 2 tablespoons of maple syrup while whisking ingredients together.

CREAMY PEANUT BUTTER OATS

DAIRY-FREE, GLUTEN-FREE, VEGAN
YIELDS 1 TO 2 CUPS

Oats are one of our favorite ingredients to have on hand for a hearty breakfast in minutes. In this recipe, oats act as a great base for introducing peanut or other nut butters. You can also use fortified baby oatmeal for a smoother texture. This recipe makes more than a baby will eat in one sitting, so plan to share this breakfast with the rest of the family.

1 cup water
½ cup old-fashioned oats

1 tablespoon creamy peanut butter
1 tablespoon coconut oil

½ teaspoon vanilla extract
1 very ripe banana, mashed (optional)

1. In a medium saucepan, bring the water to a boil. Add the oats and return to a boil, then reduce heat to low and cover.

2. Cook until the desired texture is reached. Stir in the peanut butter, coconut oil, vanilla, and mashed banana (if using). Serve warm.

3. Refrigerate leftovers in a sealed container for up to 3 days.

TIP: Soaking oats overnight in water helps break down their phytic acid, making them easier to digest and allowing for better absorption of minerals. To make even creamier oats just for baby, substitute breast milk or formula for water.

CINNAMON FRIED APPLES

GLUTEN-FREE, NUT-FREE, VEGETARIAN
YIELDS ABOUT 2 CUPS

Apples have an amazing way of becoming sweet and caramel-like when pan-fried. This recipe is quick and easy but feels like such a treat. Serve with plain Greek yogurt for breakfast, or alongside pork or chicken for dinner. Substitute coconut oil for butter to make them dairy-free.

4 tablespoons butter or coconut oil

4 apples, peeled, cored, and thinly sliced

1 teaspoon cinnamon

1 teaspoon lemon juice

1. In a large skillet over medium heat, melt the butter and swirl to coat the pan. Add the sliced apples, cinnamon, and lemon juice, and cook for 10 to 15 minutes, stirring and flipping apples every 3 minutes.

2. Refrigerate leftovers in a sealed container for up to 3 days.

TIP: Blend with some plain yogurt and a splash of milk for a delicious apple pie-flavored smoothie.

BLUEBERRY SMOOTHIE BOWL

FREEZER-FRIENDLY, GLUTEN-FREE, NUT-FREE, VEGETARIAN
YIELDS ABOUT 1 TO 2 CUPS

This yogurt- and fruit-based smoothie bowl is thick and creamy, making it the perfect consistency for self-feeding and utensil practice. Spoon it right onto your baby's tray or use a preloaded spoon.

½ ripe avocado
1 frozen banana

½ cup blueberries, fresh or frozen

½ cup plain whole milk Greek yogurt

1. Place all ingredients in a food processor and blend until smooth and creamy. Serve immediately.

2. Freeze leftovers in ice pop molds for up to 3 months.

HAPPY BELLY SMOOTHIE

FREEZER-FRIENDLY, DAIRY-FREE, GLUTEN-FREE, VEGAN
YIELDS 1¾ CUPS

When beginning solids, some babies experience occasional constipation. We've got you covered if you have an uncomfortable baby—the combination of peaches, prunes, dates, and flaxseed in this recipe has a natural laxative effect that is mild enough to include this smoothie regularly in your baby's diet.

½ cup frozen peaches
2 Medjool dates, pitted
2 prunes

1 cup almond milk
1 tablespoon
ground flaxseed

½ teaspoon
cinnamon (optional)

1. Combine all ingredients in a blender and process until smooth, about 60 seconds. Serve immediately.

2. Leftover smoothie can be poured into empty ice pop molds and frozen for up to 3 months.

TIP: Many pediatricians have come up with unique whole food ideas for easing constipation. If you find the problem is frequent or persistent, give your pediatrician's office a call.

WHOLE FRUIT GUMMIES

DAIRY-FREE, GLUTEN-FREE, NUT-FREE
YIELDS 3½ CUPS

Making your own gummies might sound intimidating, but it is surprisingly simple. The texture is closer to gelatin than the packaged treats. Subtly sweetened with whole fruit, these gummies are a treat your family will surely enjoy.

2 cups frozen blackberries, raspberries, blueberries, strawberries, or cherries

4 (2¼-teaspoon) packets unflavored gelatin
1 cup cold water

½ cup 100% fruit juice or water
1 teaspoon vanilla extract

1. Thaw the frozen berries in the refrigerator.

2. Line a 9-by-13-inch baking dish with parchment paper.

3. In a small bowl, combine the gelatin packets with 1 cup cold water and allow it to thicken for about 5 minutes.

4. In a blender, add the thawed berries, juice, and vanilla, and blend until smooth.

5. Pour the berry mixture into a saucepan, and heat over medium heat until warmed through. Add the gelatin mixture into the warm berry mixture, and stir until the gelatin is dissolved.

6. Remove from heat and let cool for 15 to 20 minutes. Pour into the prepared baking dish and refrigerate until set, about 2 hours.

7. Once set, cut gummies into thin strips for younger babies. For older babies, cut into small squares or use cookie cutters to create fun shapes.

8. Store in a sealed container in the refrigerator for up to 1 week.

TIP: If you would like a very smooth texture, strain the mixture to remove seeds and pulp before adding the gelatin.

BANANA-AVOCADO TEETHING ICE POPS

FREEZER-FRIENDLY, GLUTEN-FREE, NUT-FREE, VEGETARIAN
YIELDS 6 SMALL ICE POPS

These nutrient-rich, high-calorie freezer pops are a great snack for a teething baby who may be temporarily uninterested in eating. The mixture is also tasty on its own before freezing. For a sweeter pop, try using vanilla Greek yogurt.

1 very ripe banana
1 ripe avocado

½ cup plain whole milk
Greek yogurt

1. Combine all ingredients in a food processor and blend until smooth and creamy.

2. Using a rubber spatula, scoop the mixture out of the blender into ice pop molds or small paper cups. If using paper cups, cover each cup with tin foil and press a baby spoon or self-feeding utensil through the foil into the mixture.

3. Freeze until solid, about 6 hours or overnight. If using paper cups, peel off the paper cup and remove foil once frozen.

4. Store in the freezer for up to 3 months.

TIP: There are a few ice pop molds on the market just for babies, featuring easy-to-grip handles and small serving sizes. Nuby and Zoku both offer a variety of options (available on Amazon).

WHOLE FRUIT SOFT SERVE

FREEZER-FRIENDLY, DAIRY-FREE, GLUTEN-FREE, NUT-FREE, VEGAN
YIELDS 4 (½-CUP) SERVINGS

This creamy soft serve has just two ingredients: whole fruit and a splash of coconut milk. Use whatever frozen fruit you have on hand. Coconut milk makes this treat extra creamy, but other types of milk will work as well.

1 (16-ounce) bag frozen fruit (like strawberries, peaches, mango, or pineapple)

⅓ cup full-fat coconut milk

1. Combine the frozen fruit and coconut milk in a food processor. Process until smooth, stopping as needed to scrape down the sides.

2. Serve immediately for a smooth, soft-serve-like consistency, or freeze in a sealed container for up to 3 months. If frozen, let thaw for about 15 minutes before serving to make it soft enough to scoop.

TIP: If you would like a sweeter "ice cream," add 1 frozen ripe banana to the food processor before blending.

WARM SPICED CARROT-PEAR SAUCE

FREEZER-FRIENDLY, DAIRY-FREE, GLUTEN-FREE, NUT-FREE, VEGAN
YIELDS ABOUT 10 (½-CUP) SERVINGS

The idea for this pear sauce came from an overabundance of pears from Laura's tree one fall. It's remarkable how sweet this sauce is from the fruit alone, and it is a fave of our little ones. We eat it like applesauce, and it's very versatile. Use it to sweeten oatmeal, substitute it for applesauce in baking, serve it as a side dish, or use it as a dip for cinnamon toast. Bonus: These spices will make your house smell amazing.

10 pears or apples, peeled, cored, and chopped

3 large carrots, peeled and chopped

2 teaspoons cinnamon

1 teaspoon ground ginger

½ teaspoon nutmeg

¼ teaspoon cloves

1. Combine all ingredients in a slow cooker. Cook on high for 5 to 6 hours, until soft.

2. Purée in batches in a food processor or blender. You can also use an immersion blender right in the slow cooker. If using a blender, open the center of the lid to prevent steam buildup, and cover the opening with a towel while blending (hot liquid may splatter if you don't!).

3. Store sauce in a sealed container in the refrigerator for a week, or freeze up to 3 months. Thaw in refrigerator overnight if frozen.

TIP: Try offering this sweet sauce alongside tart plain yogurt. This recipe is also great for use in baking, like in our Autumn-Spiced Apple Donuts (page 131).

PEANUT BUTTER MOUSSE

GLUTEN-FREE, VEGETARIAN
YIELDS ½ CUP

This is one of our favorite ways to introduce peanut butter, which is rich in protein and healthy fat. As your baby gets used to peanut butter, feel free to add in more, but just make sure it is blended well. Keep in mind that in addition to peanut butter, this recipe includes milk, another top allergen, so we recommend offering this recipe after you've determined that your baby tolerates dairy. Regular and Greek yogurt both work well in this recipe.

½ cup plain or vanilla whole milk yogurt

2 teaspoons creamy peanut butter

1. In a small bowl, whisk together the yogurt and peanut butter until smooth and creamy.

2. Serve immediately.

TIP: Try offering this mousse as a dip for soft fruit. For toddlers, stir in a teaspoon of maple syrup or a swirl of mini chocolate chips for a protein-packed dessert.

BAKED ZUCCHINI FINGERS

NUT-FREE, VEGETARIAN
YIELDS 4 SERVINGS

One of Laura's favorite foods growing up, especially in the summer months, was fried zucchini. This oven-baked treat will easily become a favorite side dish for your family as well. Serve with low-sodium marinara sauce for dipping, if desired.

½ cup panko breadcrumbs

2 tablespoons shredded or grated Parmesan cheese

½ teaspoon garlic powder

1 teaspoon basil

1 teaspoon oregano

3 medium zucchini

2 eggs

¼ cup milk

1. Preheat the oven to 400°F. Line a rimmed baking sheet with parchment paper.

2. Place the breadcrumbs, cheese, garlic powder, basil, and oregano in a large container with a tight-fitting lid or a zip-top bag, and shake well to combine.

3. Cut the zucchini in half and then into thin strips.

4. In a shallow dish, beat the egg and milk until well combined. Dip the zucchini strips one at a time into the egg and milk mixture, then into the breadcrumb mixture, then lay them on the prepared baking sheet, spreading them evenly.

5. Bake for 15 minutes or until lightly browned.

6. Refrigerate leftovers in a sealed container for up to 3 days, and pop in the toaster oven to reheat.

CARROT FRIES

DAIRY-FREE, GLUTEN-FREE, NUT-FREE, VEGAN
YIELDS ABOUT 3 CUPS

Carrots are one of the most inexpensive, nutrition-packed produce items in the grocery store. Delicious and filled with beta-carotene, fiber, and vitamin K, carrots get you plenty of crunch for your buck. For infant and toddler safety, *always* cut carrots lengthwise and roast or steam them until they are nice and soft.

8 large carrots, cut into matchsticks (see Tip)

2 tablespoons extra-virgin olive oil

2 teaspoons smoked paprika

1. Preheat the oven to 375°F. Line a baking sheet with parchment paper.

2. Place the carrots, olive oil, and paprika in a mixing bowl or zip-top bag, and toss until coated.

3. Spread carrots in a single layer on the prepared baking sheet. Bake for about 35 minutes, or until desired tenderness, flipping halfway through.

4. Store leftovers in a covered container in the refrigerator. For best results, reheat in the oven.

TIP: To cut carrots into matchsticks, wash and scrub the carrots with a vegetable brush (peeling is optional). Cut off the ends of the carrots, then slice them in half lengthwise. Lay the carrot halves on their flat sides, and then cut them into thirds, until they are the width of a pencil, then cut the long strips in half so they are the size of French fries. Use this matchstick cut-and-roast method on any of your favorite vegetables—or make a colorful veggie medley with orange and purple carrots and parsnips! Try dipping them in our Easy Tzatziki Sauce (page 100).

LENTIL FRITTERS

FREEZER-FRIENDLY, NUT-FREE, VEGETARIAN
YIELDS 10 TO 15 FRITTERS

Lentils are naturally packed with protein, iron, and fiber, making them an ideal ingredient for your infant's diet. Their versatility lends them to soups or salads, or use them as a filler in meatloaf or fritters like these.

1 cup red or green split lentils, soaked 3 to 4 hours in water, rinsed, and drained

1 cup minced baby kale, spinach, or dark greens of choice

1 cup grated sweet potato or 1 large baked and cooled sweet potato

1 egg

¼ cup grated Parmesan cheese

1 teaspoon minced garlic

¼ teaspoon cumin

¼ teaspoon finely chopped onion

¼ teaspoon paprika

¼ teaspoon salt

½ cup quick-cook or old-fashioned oats

2 tablespoons extra-virgin olive oil

1. Line your work surface with parchment paper.

2. In a food processor, pulse the lentils, kale, sweet potato, egg, cheese, garlic, cumin, onion, paprika, and salt together until you reach a chunky-creamy consistency.

3. Transfer the lentil mixture to a medium mixing bowl, and stir in the oats.

4. With your hands, shape the batter into thin sticks (length of middle finger and diameter of pinkie), and place on the prepared work surface.

5. In a large nonstick skillet over medium heat, heat the oil. Fry the fritters, turning to get all sides golden brown. Let cool before serving.

6. Store leftovers in a sealed container in the refrigerator for up to 3 days or freeze in a freezer-safe container. Pop them in the oven for a quick side or snack.

ROASTED CAULIFLOWER STEAKS

FREEZER-FRIENDLY, GLUTEN-FREE, NUT-FREE, VEGETARIAN
YIELDS 6 LARGE SLICES

Cauliflower is a great food to include in a baby's early days because it becomes very tender and flavorful when roasted. Some people are surprised to find out how nutrient-packed cauliflower is. Despite its pale color, it is a tremendously antioxidant-rich vegetable.

Oil or butter, for greasing

1 large head cauliflower

3 tablespoons extra-virgin olive oil

½ teaspoon dried thyme

½ teaspoon dried rosemary

½ teaspoon garlic powder

¼ cup shredded Parmesan cheese

1. Preheat the oven to 400°F. Lightly grease a rimmed baking sheet, or line with parchment paper.

2. Slice the cauliflower into 1-inch-thick steaks and lay flat on the prepared baking sheet. Drizzle with olive oil and sprinkle seasonings on top. Move the steaks around on baking sheet to ensure each one is covered on all sides with oil and seasoning.

3. Bake for about 25 minutes, until the cauliflower is lightly brown and very tender. Remove from the oven and top with cheese. Let cool slightly and break into finger-length florets to serve.

4. Store leftovers in the refrigerator for 2 to 3 days, or freeze in a sealed container for up to 3 months.

TIP: Leftover veggies like these are great with breakfast the next day.

SO-GOOD GUACAMOLE

DAIRY-FREE, NUT-FREE, GLUTEN-FREE, VEGAN
YIELDS 2 CUPS

This recipe is very versatile. Consider making two batches—if your family likes the heat, throw in some more cumin or even a pinch of cayenne pepper in one of them. For your baby, serve this guacamole on a preloaded spoon, spread on strips of soft toast, or mashed with black beans; for adults and older kids, serve with tortilla chips or carrot sticks.

3 or 4 ripe avocados
1 tomato, diced
½ medium red onion, finely chopped

1 tablespoon lime juice
1 teaspoon cumin
½ teaspoon salt

¼ teaspoon freshly ground black pepper

1. Place each avocado lengthwise on a cutting surface, and use a sharp knife to slice through the skin and around the large pit.

2. Twist to separate the halves. With a large metal spoon, carefully remove the pit, then scoop the flesh into a bowl. Discard the skins and pits.

3. Gently mash the avocado flesh with a fork or potato masher until a creamy, chunky balance is reached.

4. Add the remaining ingredients and mix until just combined. Season with additional spices to taste.

5. Serve immediately.

TIP: Avocados brown quickly, so this is not a good "meal prep" side dish. Just remember to prepare this right before serving—it can be mashed up in minutes. Leftovers may be stored in the refrigerator in a dish covered with plastic wrap touching the avocado to prevent oxidation. Scrape off the brown top layer before serving again the next day.

NUTTY MASHED SWEET POTATOES

DAIRY-FREE, GLUTEN-FREE, VEGAN
YIELDS 2 (½-CUP) SERVINGS

Sweet potatoes quickly became a go-to when we were giving first foods to our kids. They are very soft, naturally sweet, and packed with nutrients. The sweet side is enhanced with creamy cashew butter and spicy cinnamon.

1 large sweet potato, roasted or boiled
2 tablespoons cashew butter
1 tablespoon coconut oil
1 teaspoon cinnamon

1. Remove the sweet potato flesh from the skin, and mash with the cashew butter, coconut oil, and cinnamon until smooth. Let the mixture cool to room temperature.

2. Serve on a preloaded spoon.

3. Store leftovers in the refrigerator for up to 2 days.

TIP: Swap out the cashew butter for almond or peanut butter for a change in flavor and texture and exposure to different allergens. If your grocer carries them, you can also try using yellow or purple sweet potatoes instead of the typical orange-fleshed varieties.

TWO-INGREDIENT SWEET POTATO TORTILLAS

FREEZER-FRIENDLY, NUT-FREE, VEGAN
YIELDS 12 SMALL TORTILLAS

Making tortillas at home is incredibly quick and easy, thanks to this two-ingredient recipe (three if you count the oil). The result is a soft, pliable wrap that's perfect for handheld breakfast burritos, quesadillas, or tacos. Sprinkle with a little coarse salt right after frying if desired. Slice them into strips or offer your baby a whole one.

2 cups unbleached all-purpose flour

1½ cups mashed cooked sweet potato

2 tablespoons coconut oil, divided, plus more if needed

1. In a medium bowl, use a spoon or floured hands to combine the flour and sweet potato until a soft dough forms. If the dough is sticky, add in more flour, 1 tablespoon at a time. The dough should be soft but not sticky.

2. Separate the dough into 12 equal balls. Dust your work surface with flour, and use a rolling pin to roll out each ball into ¼-inch thick tortillas.

3. In a skillet over medium heat, add 1 tablespoon of coconut oil (or enough to fully coat the bottom of the pan). Fry the tortillas, 1 or 2 at a time, for about 1 minute on each side, adding more coconut oil as needed every few batches. Serve warm.

4. Refrigerate any extras in a sealed container with parchment paper in between each tortilla for up to 3 days. Freeze in a zip-top bag with parchment paper in between each tortilla for up to 3 months.

TIP: Try adding fresh or dried herbs to the dough before forming the tortillas. Garlic and rosemary are family favorites!

SWEET POTATO AND RED ONION FRITTATA WITH KALE AND GOAT CHEESE

GLUTEN-FREE, NUT-FREE, VEGETARIAN
YIELDS 1 (12-INCH) FRITTATA

Three reasons we love this recipe: It features three different vegetables; it's great for breakfast, lunch, or dinner; and it's ready to eat in 30 minutes—hands-on time is more like 15. Roasting the veggie mixture before stirring in the eggs ensures everything is nice and tender. We recommend a cast-iron skillet for this recipe, but any ovenproof skillet will do.

3 medium sweet potatoes, peeled and chopped

1 large red onion, chopped

4 tablespoons extra-virgin olive oil, divided

Salt

Freshly ground black pepper

3 cups baby kale, chopped

12 eggs, beaten

6 ounces goat cheese, crumbled

1. Preheat the oven to 425°F. Toss the sweet potatoes and red onion with 2 tablespoons of olive oil, sprinkle with salt and pepper, and roast until cooked through, about 25 minutes.

2. In a 12-inch cast-iron skillet over medium heat, heat the remaining 2 tablespoons of olive oil. Add the baby kale and sauté for a few minutes.

3. Add the roasted potato mixture and beaten eggs to the skillet, stirring quickly to combine. Then cook without stirring for 2 minutes, or until the edges start to set.

4. Sprinkle in the crumbled goat cheese, and transfer to the oven. Bake for 10 to 15 more minutes, until the frittata is set in the center. Slice into strips and serve.

5. Refrigerate leftovers in a sealed container for up to 3 days.

AVOCADO EGG SALAD

GLUTEN-FREE, NUT-FREE, VEGETARIAN
YIELDS 4 SERVINGS

This twist on traditional egg salad packs a punch with choline, protein, and healthy fat. It's delicious on its own or spread on strips of toast. Also, when it comes to feeding bread to babies, you don't always have to go whole grain. Little ones have little tummies and fill up very quickly on fiber-rich foods. Aim to use whole grains about half the time.

2 ripe avocados

2 teaspoons fresh lemon juice

4 tablespoons plain Greek yogurt

2 tablespoons chopped cilantro

6 hard boiled eggs, peeled and finely chopped

1. Halve the avocados, remove the pits, and scoop the flesh into a large bowl.

2. Mash the avocado with the lemon juice. Add the Greek yogurt and cilantro, and mix well. Stir in the chopped eggs and mix until combined.

3. Refrigerate leftovers in a sealed container for up to 2 days.

CREAMY TOMATO SOUP

FREEZER-FRIENDLY, DAIRY-FREE, GLUTEN-FREE, NUT-FREE, VEGAN
YIELDS 4 CUPS

Chickpeas are blended into this tomato soup, giving it a thick, creamy texture that's easy for infants to get onto a spoon or even scoop with their hands (be careful not to serve this soup too hot!). Serve with strips of toast for dipping.

2 tablespoons extra-virgin olive oil

1 small onion, diced

4 garlic cloves, diced

1 (28-ounce) can low-sodium diced or crushed tomatoes

½ cup low-sodium vegetable stock

1½ cups canned chickpeas, drained and rinsed

½ teaspoon oregano

1. In a stockpot or Dutch oven over medium heat, heat the olive oil until it shimmers. Add the diced onion and cook, stirring occasionally, until softened. Add the garlic and cook, stirring frequently for a minute or two or until fragrant.

2. Pour in the tomatoes and vegetable stock. Stir in the chickpeas. Sprinkle in the oregano, cover, and let simmer for about 15 minutes.

3. Blend the soup with an immersion blender until smooth, or in batches in a food processor.

4. Let cool to a warm temperature, and top with coarse salt before serving.

5. Refrigerate leftovers in a sealed container for up to 3 days.

TIP: This soup makes a nutrient-packed dip or spread; it goes especially well with our Baked Zucchini Fingers (page 66).

BASIC BLACK BEANS

DAIRY-FREE, GLUTEN-FREE, NUT-FREE, VEGAN
YIELDS 3 CUPS

Beans are such a versatile ingredient and, arguably, one of the most nutrient-packed foods on earth, full of protein, iron, and fiber—a winning nutrient combination in BLW. Unfortunately, while working as registered dietitians in schools, we learned that many children are unfamiliar with beans, and, therefore, many older children are unwilling to give them a try. We want to change that by making kids fans at a young age.

1 (15.5-ounce) can black beans, or 1 cup dried beans, soaked overnight, then rinsed

½ cup finely chopped onion

2 garlic cloves, minced

1 teaspoon cumin

1. For canned beans: In a small saucepan on medium-high heat, combine the beans, onion, garlic, and cumin. Bring to a boil for at least 5 minutes, then simmer on low heat for 30 minutes, or until the onion and garlic are completely cooked through. If the beans begin to look dry, add water or low-sodium broth, a few tablespoons at a time.

2. For dried beans: In a large stockpot, bring 4 cups water to a boil. Add the beans and return to a boil for a few minutes. Reduce heat to a simmer. Add the onion, garlic, and cumin. Allow to simmer, covered, for 1½ to 2 hours, until desired tenderness is reached. If the beans begin to look dry, add water or low-sodium broth, ¼ cup at a time, until desired consistency is achieved.

3. Store leftovers in a sealed container in the refrigerator for up to 3 days.

TIP: These basic beans can be paired with many recipes. They're a great side to the Easy Tuna Quesadilla (page 122), or you can even drain and wrap the beans inside it.

BLACK BEAN HUMMUS

DAIRY-FREE, GLUTEN-FREE, VEGAN
YIELDS ABOUT 2 CUPS

Packed with iron and antioxidants, beans are a great protein source. Offer them to your baby at least a few times a week. For this twist on the traditional chick-pea dish, we've added tart and tangy Kalamata olives—it's never too early to introduce your baby to the world of savory treats! Serve this dip with very thin strips of bell pepper or cucumber, or use as a topping for crackers or toast. You can also offer it on a preloaded spoon.

1 (15-ounce) can black beans, drained, liquid reserved (or use Basic Black Beans, page 76)

1 clove garlic, finely chopped, or 1 teaspoon garlic powder

2 tablespoons lemon juice

1½ tablespoons tahini

½ teaspoon salt

½ teaspoon ground cumin (optional)

¼ teaspoon paprika, plus more for garnish

⅛ teaspoon cayenne pepper (optional)

10 sliced Kalamata olives, for garnish

1. In a food processor, combine all the ingredients except the olives. Pulse and then scrape down the sides of the processor. Pulse again, then spoon into a serving bowl. Garnish with paprika and olives.

2. Refrigerate leftovers in a sealed container for up to 3 days.

BLACK BEAN BURGERS

FREEZER-FRIENDLY, DAIRY-FREE, VEGETARIAN
YIELDS 6 BURGER PATTIES

Try this bold vegetarian burger, featuring nutrition-packed and hearty black beans, almonds, and breadcrumbs. Rich in iron and fiber, these can be served alone, with a mashed avocado to dip, or assembled like a traditional burger. For parents or older children, give them a Tex-Mex spin with sliced Monterey Jack cheese, our So-Good Guacamole (page 70), and a tomato slice, all on a grilled bun.

4 tablespoons extra-virgin olive oil, divided
½ medium onion, diced
⅓ cup roasted almonds

1¾ cups Basic Black Beans (page 76)
⅔ cup whole-wheat panko breadcrumbs

1 egg, lightly beaten
1 teaspoon smoked paprika
Salt
Freshly ground black pepper

1. In a skillet over medium heat, heat 1 tablespoon of olive oil. Sauté the diced onion until it is translucent, about 5 minutes. Remove from the heat.

2. In a food processor, pulse the almonds until fine crumbs form. Add the cooked onion, black beans, breadcrumbs, egg, and paprika, and pulse until combined. Season with salt and black pepper.

3. Transfer the mixture to a bowl and mix well. Form into 6 patties. In a medium skillet over medium heat, heat the remaining 3 tablespoons olive oil. Cook the patties, flipping once, until lightly browned and crispy on both sides.

4. Store leftovers in a sealed container in the refrigerator for 2 to 3 days. To freeze, place patties in a freezer-safe container with parchment paper between each patty.

TIP: The almonds in this recipe add a nice toasty flavor, but you can substitute an additional ⅓ cup breadcrumbs in their place.

QUINOA TURKEY MINI MEATBALLS

FREEZER-FRIENDLY, DAIRY-FREE, GLUTEN-FREE, NUT-FREE
YIELDS ABOUT 25 MEATBALLS

These quick and easy meatballs are high in both iron and protein, and the apple adds a touch of sweetness little ones love. They freeze well, making them the perfect addition to your meal prep routine.

1 pound ground turkey	2 eggs, lightly beaten	1 teaspoon garlic powder
2 cups cooked quinoa	2 tablespoons tomato paste	1 teaspoon dried oregano
1 apple, peeled and grated	1 teaspoon chopped fresh or dried basil	3 tablespoons extra-virgin olive oil

1. Preheat the oven to 350°F. Line a rimmed baking sheet with parchment paper.

2. In a large bowl, combine the turkey, quinoa, apple, eggs, tomato paste, basil, garlic powder, and oregano until well mixed. Use a 1-tablespoon measuring spoon to scoop the mixture, and roll each scoop into a mini meatball. Place each meatball a few inches apart on the prepared baking sheet.

3. Drizzle the meatballs with the olive oil and bake for about 30 minutes, or until they reach an interior temperature of at least 165°F. Let rest for a few minutes before serving.

4. Store leftover cooked meatballs in a sealed container in the refrigerator for 2 to 3 days.

TIP: If you're planning to freeze this recipe, *do not cook the meatballs*. Form meatballs on a lined baking sheet, and place in the freezer for a few hours until firm. Remove the frozen meatballs and transfer to a zip-top freezer bag. Freeze for up to 3 months. To cook, place frozen meatballs on a prepared baking sheet (do not thaw), and follow the baking instructions, adding about 15 minutes to the cooking time.

SLOW COOKER CHICKEN WITH PEANUT SAUCE

FREEZER-FRIENDLY, DAIRY-FREE
YIELDS 8 CHICKEN THIGHS

This recipe is on an almost-weekly rotation in our homes. Slow-cooked chicken, especially dark meat, is a great choice during the first few weeks of baby-led weaning. Not only is it incredibly tender when cooked this way, it's high in easily absorbed iron. Try this dish over quinoa or rice, with roasted carrots on the side.

1 cup full-fat coconut milk

⅓ cup creamy peanut butter

3 tablespoons brown sugar

1 tablespoon reduced-sodium soy sauce

1 tablespoon apple cider vinegar

1 teaspoon garlic powder

½ teaspoon ground ginger

1½ pounds boneless, skinless chicken thighs

Fresh cilantro for topping (optional)

1. In a 6-quart slow cooker, add the coconut milk, peanut butter, brown sugar, soy sauce, vinegar, garlic powder, and ginger. Whisk together to make a sauce.

2. Top the sauce with the chicken in a single layer, spooning some of the sauce over the chicken to coat. Cook on high for 4 to 5 hours. Chicken should fall off the bone and be easily shredded with a fork.

3. Serve topped with cilantro (if using).

4. Store leftover chicken in a sealed container in the refrigerator for 2 to 3 days. Freeze leftovers in a sealed container or zip-top freezer bag for up to 3 months.

TIP: Most soy sauce contains wheat. If you want your sauce to be gluten-free, substitute tamari, which typically only contains soy; however, make sure you check the label, as not all brands are certified gluten-free.

LEMON BUTTER SHEET PAN SHRIMP

GLUTEN-FREE, NUT-FREE
YIELDS 20 TO 24 SHRIMP

Sheet pan dinners are lifesavers during a busy workweek for their easy prep and quick cleanup. This recipe is a fun way to introduce your baby to shellfish, a common allergen. Plus, shrimp is great for self-feeding because it naturally comes with a convenient little handle, which is perfect for babies.

Extra-virgin olive oil, for greasing the pan

½ cup butter, melted

4 garlic cloves, minced

1 tablespoon lemon juice

½ teaspoon Italian seasoning

¼ teaspoon salt

⅛ teaspoon freshly ground black pepper

1½ pounds large shrimp, peeled, deveined, and butterflied

2 tablespoons chopped fresh parsley (optional)

Sliced lemons (optional)

1. Preheat oven to 400°F. Lightly grease a rimmed sheet pan with olive oil.

2. In a medium bowl, whisk together the melted butter, garlic, lemon juice, Italian seasoning, salt, and pepper.

3. Add the shrimp to the mixture and gently toss to combine. Spread the shrimp in a single layer on the prepared baking sheet.

4. Bake until the shrimp begin to firm and turn slightly pink, 8 to 10 minutes.

5. Garnish with parsley and/or sliced lemons (if using). Serve warm with shrimp sliced lengthwise.

6. Refrigerate leftovers in a sealed container for up to 2 days.

TIP: For a complete meal with easy cleanup, use a larger sheet pan and throw on some fresh veggies to roast alongside the protein. Broccoli or asparagus both taste great with this citrus Italian marinade. Veggies may need more bake time than the tender shrimp, so start those for 10 minutes, then throw on the shrimp.

SALMON CAKES

NUT-FREE

YIELDS ABOUT 10 (3-OUNCE) PATTIES

These salmon cakes are a great midweek, high-protein meal that requires minimal prep and no thawing time. This recipe is a staple in our kitchens and helps us meet our goal of eating fish twice a week.

1 (14.75-ounce) can salmon, drained and flaked

½ cup Italian breadcrumbs or crushed crackers, such as Ritz or saltines

¼ cup minced fresh parsley

1 egg, beaten

½ onion, diced

1½ teaspoons freshly ground black pepper

1½ teaspoons garlic powder

3 tablespoons grated Parmesan cheese

1 tablespoon Dijon mustard

1 tablespoon lemon or lime juice

3 tablespoons extra-virgin olive oil, plus more as needed

1. In a large bowl, mix together the salmon, breadcrumbs, parsley, egg, onion, black pepper, garlic powder, cheese, mustard, and lemon juice.

2. Divide and shape the mixture into approximately 10 patties.

3. In a large skillet over medium heat, add the olive oil and swirl to cover the pan. In batches, fry the salmon patties until browned, 4 to 5 minutes per side. Add more olive oil as needed. Let cool slightly before serving.

4. Store leftovers in the refrigerator and reheat in the oven for best quality.

TIP: Look for salmon without bones, or carefully remove the bones before serving. For older toddlers (about 18 months and up), the bones are actually safely edible and a great source of calcium.

**BETTER-THAN-BOXED
MACARONI AND CHEESE**
PAGE 157

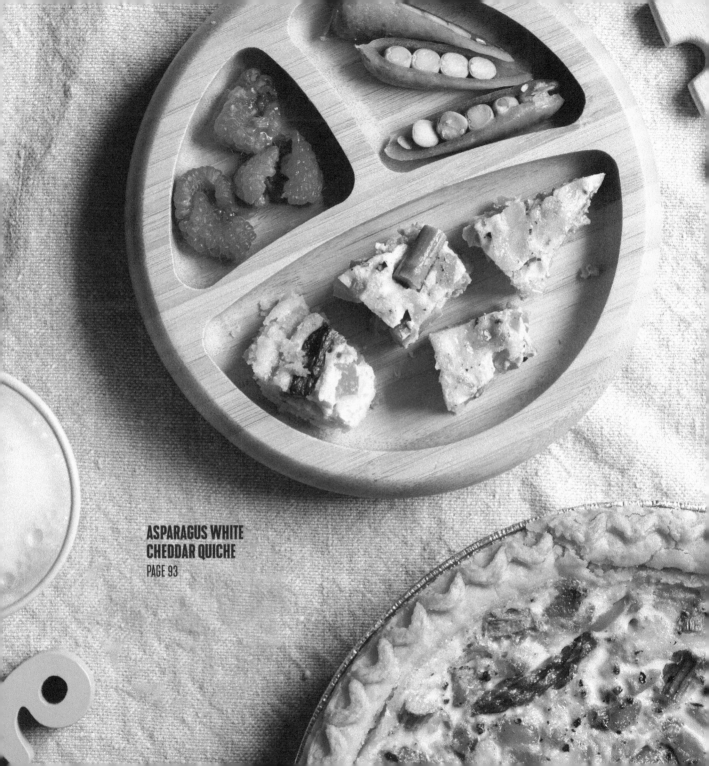

**ASPARAGUS WHITE
CHEDDAR QUICHE**
PAGE 93

CHAPTER 4
9 TO 12 MONTHS
NEW TEXTURES AND FLAVORS

WHAT TO EXPECT

In the blink of an eye, your sweet, tiny, innocent newborn baby is now moving, crawling, stumbling, and maybe even walking. Touching, throwing, pulling, poking, pinching, and very much intentionally dropping. Babbling, always slobbering, exclaiming, naming, and maybe even signing. Yelling, shouting, singing, and most importantly, confidently self-feeding!

This window of time is often the sweet spot in BLW because babies are feeding well but also still very accepting of new foods. Take advantage of this period and introduce as many ingredients, flavors, and textures as possible.

If you are practicing mealtime baby sign language, you may notice your child signing back a few key phrases. Continue to speak and sign with them as you add to your signing repertoire. With their newfound mobility and independence, mealtime expectations are about to be put to the test. Remember that section on the importance of family mealtimes? This is a good time to reread it (page 37)!

Baby's Motor Skills

During these months, physical, mental, social, and emotional development is progressing at the speed of light. In addition to a strong hand grasp, your child will now begin to use the pincer grasp (thumb and index finger) to pick up smaller foods like halved or quartered berries, green peas, semi-mashed beans, dry cereals, cut olives, and hopefully even their own crumbs.

Continue to offer self-feeding utensils, although babies at this age still tend to prefer their hands. However, they may begin experimenting with utensils, especially if introduced right from the start.

Eating at This Stage

In this stage, you can increase from two to three meals per day, but do what feels right for your family. You might be getting the hang of portion sizes that work for your baby. Offer as much food as they want, paying close attention to requests for more. Babies are great self-regulators and may be eating more in response to a growth spurt or developmental leap.

Most of your baby's nutrient needs are still being met with breast milk or formula. Try offering the breast or bottle following meals or snacks rather than beforehand—your baby is beginning to understand the expectations of self-feeding and can sit down to a meal a little hungry. Continue breast- or bottle-feeding on demand or on a schedule.

Recipes at This Stage

The recipes in this section combine different textures and flavors, while keeping a focus on important nutrients like iron, calories, and fat. These recipes also have a few more ingredients and spices/seasonings to experiment with.

If you haven't attempted spices with your baby yet, give it a try. Exposure to a variety of flavors can help a baby grow to accept more foods. The recipes in this section contain a variety of spices and herbs to try. However, you won't find a lot of added salt. If you are sharing the meal, adults can add salt to their own serving at the table.

Try offering a variety of sizes and shapes of food, like diced pieces. Your little one will soon be able to pick up small pieces efficiently with that pincer grasp they're working on. They may also be mastering utensils, making foods like soups and dips (hopefully) a little less messy. Make sure you continue to focus on a variety of textures to support long-term acceptance.

As your baby gets more teeth, they may begin to bite off larger pieces of food. Most of the time, if a baby bites off a piece of food that is uncomfortably large, they will spit it out or gag it to the front of the mouth.

To alleviate any fears that they'll bite off too large a chunk, you can offer very small pieces of food like meat or veggies once a pincer grasp is present. You can also consider offering a much larger piece for them to gnaw on for firmer foods like steak as you supervise. Keep in mind that the large bites we take as adults often require our molars, so a baby will have a hard time removing a big chunk. But eventually, your child will get it, so always be on the lookout.

Now, let's take our new skills to the table!

LIGHT AND AIRY BANANA BREAD BITES

FREEZER-FRIENDLY, NUT-FREE, VEGETARIAN
YIELDS 24 MINI MUFFINS

These little muffins are sweetened with banana, so there's no need for added sugar. They can be made using just one bowl, which is a major win in our book! Try mixing in some very finely chopped walnuts or mini chocolate chips for a change.

Butter for greasing the pan

1 large, very ripe banana (½ cup mashed)

½ cup milk

2 teaspoons apple cider vinegar

2 teaspoons vanilla extract

3 tablespoons coconut oil, melted

¾ cup unbleached all-purpose flour

½ teaspoon baking powder

½ teaspoon baking soda

½ teaspoon cinnamon

1. Preheat the oven to 350°F. Butter a mini muffin tin.

2. In a large bowl, mash the banana with the milk. Stir in the vinegar, vanilla, and melted coconut oil, and mix until well combined.

3. Add the flour, baking powder, baking soda, and cinnamon, and mix until combined.

4. Pour into the greased mini muffin tin and bake for 10 to 15 minutes, or until tops spring back when touched.

5. Serve or store. Refrigerate in a container with a tightly fitting lid for up to 3 days. Freeze baked muffins in a freezer-safe container for up to 3 months.

WARM CINNAMON BREAKFAST QUINOA

GLUTEN-FREE, NUT-FREE, VEGETARIAN
YIELDS 3 CUPS

Quinoa is packed with all nine essential amino acids, making it a complete protein. Its texture is unique and a great one to introduce to babes at a young age. This warm, sweet dish is especially convenient if you have leftover quinoa on hand!

1 tablespoon coconut oil or butter

½ teaspoon cinnamon

1 cup cooked quinoa, cooled

½ cup milk, plus more if desired

½ teaspoon vanilla extract

1 tablespoon maple syrup (optional)

1. In a small saucepan over medium-low heat, melt the coconut oil and sprinkle with cinnamon. Stir in the quinoa and milk, and cook for about 3 minutes, stirring frequently.

2. Remove from heat and stir in the vanilla. Top with the maple syrup (if using), and additional milk if desired.

3. Serve immediately, making sure it isn't too hot.

4. Store leftovers in the refrigerator for up to 2 days. Reheat in the microwave or a saucepan over medium-low heat.

TIP: To make this recipe dairy-free and vegan, use a plant-based milk and use coconut oil instead of butter. You can also increase the fiber and change the flavor by adding chopped, soft fruit like peaches, pears, bananas, or berries.

SWEET POTATO TOAST THREE WAYS

GLUTEN-FREE, NUT-FREE, VEGETARIAN
YIELDS 1 SWEET POTATO (4 TO 6 SLICES)

Did you know that thinly sliced sweet potato popped into the toaster makes a surprisingly versatile and tasty base for all kinds of toppings? When it comes to baby-led weaning, we are always looking for high-calorie options for topping toast. Try one (or all three) of these options for a different take on a classic breakfast staple. Sweet potato toast also makes a terrific last-minute lunch or dinner option.

For Sweet Potato Toast

1 medium sweet potato, peeled

FOR BERRIES AND CREAM SPREAD

2 tablespoons cream cheese

½ cup strawberries, thinly sliced

Fresh mint or basil, finely chopped (optional)

FOR SESAME AVOCADO SPREAD

2 tablespoons tahini

¼ ripe avocado, smashed

FOR GREEK PITA SPREAD

2 tablespoons full-fat Greek yogurt or Easy Tzatziki Sauce (page 100)

6 Kalamata or black olives, diced

Extra-virgin olive oil

Fresh herbs like chives, cilantro, or parsley, finely chopped (optional)

1. Slice the sweet potato lengthwise into ¼-inch slices.

2. Place two slices of sweet potato in the toaster at a time. Toast until well done, about 5 minutes. You might have to toast two to three times to reach desired texture.

3. Layer with desired spread and serve immediately.

TIP: Squish the center of each toasted sweet potato slice to make sure it is nice and soft.

SWEET POTATO, SAUSAGE, AND SPINACH BREAKFAST CASSEROLE

FREEZER-FRIENDLY, NUT-FREE
YIELDS 1 (9-BY-13-INCH) CASSEROLE

This breakfast casserole is Ellen's official "Welcome-home-new-baby-and congratulations-no-more-cold-lasagna-for-breakfast" dish, and it is absolutely delicious. Although this recipe calls for a 9-by-13-inch pan, the recipe can be cut in half and baked in an 8-by-8-inch pan, so why not make a full recipe and divide it into two 8-by-8-inch pans—one to give away and one to keep? The savory sausage and spinach make it a great breakfast-for-supper option.

Oil or butter, for greasing

1 (16-ounce) package ground sausage

½ cup finely chopped onion

1 teaspoon minced garlic

1 cup fresh spinach leaves, julienned

1 teaspoon salt (optional)

½ teaspoon freshly ground black pepper

4 cups shredded sweet potatoes, skin on or off (5 to 6 medium/large sweet potatoes)

¼ cup butter, melted

1 cup shredded mild Cheddar cheese

1 cup shredded mozzarella cheese

1 (16-ounce) container cottage cheese

10 eggs, lightly beaten

1. Preheat the oven to 375°F. Lightly grease a 9-by-13-inch baking dish.

2. In a cast-iron skillet over medium heat, brown the sausage. Add the onion and garlic, and cook until the onion is translucent.

3. Add the spinach and cook until tender. Season with the salt (if using), and pepper. Remove from heat and set aside.

4. In a medium bowl, mix the sweet potato shreds and melted butter. Evenly spread the potatoes in the bottom of the prepared baking dish and pat down evenly, creating a "crust."

5. In a large bowl, combine the Cheddar, mozzarella, and cottage cheese, eggs, and semi-cooled sausage mixture, mixing well. Spoon over the sweet potato crust.

6. Bake 50 to 60 minutes, until the center is set. To prevent overbrowning, cover with aluminum foil for the last 15 minutes of bake time. Cool for 5 minutes before serving.

7. Cut and freeze leftovers in individual portions, or freeze in a smaller baking dish and thaw and reheat when desired.

TIP: White russet potatoes can be substituted for the sweet potatoes. Feel free to add other veggies, such as sliced mushrooms, when sautéing the onions and spinach.

ASPARAGUS WHITE CHEDDAR QUICHE

FREEZER-FRIENDLY, NUT-FREE
YIELDS 2 QUICHES

When asparagus goes on sale at the grocery store, we know spring is finally near. But what should you do if asparagus is not in season? Not to worry—this recipe lends itself to substitutions and improvisation. It's also a great way to clean out your crisper drawer! Try using sliced tomatoes, mushrooms, Swiss cheese, or fresh herbs.

1 pound fresh asparagus, ends trimmed, spears cut into ½-inch pieces (see Tip)

1 to 2 tablespoons extra-virgin olive oil

½ cup diced onion

½ cup diced bell pepper

1 teaspoon minced garlic

2 (8-inch) pie shells, or homemade pie crust (page 119)

1 egg white, lightly beaten

10 slices bacon, cooked and crumbled, or ½ cup real bacon bits

2 cups shredded white Cheddar cheese

6 eggs

1½ cups half-and-half

¼ teaspoon ground nutmeg

½ teaspoon salt (optional)

¼ teaspoon freshly ground black pepper

1. Preheat the oven to 400°F. (If using homemade pie crust, line two 9-inch pie plates with dough and place in the refrigerator to set into shells.)

2. In a medium skillet over medium heat, sauté the asparagus with the olive oil, onion, bell pepper, and garlic.

3. Brush the pie shells with beaten egg white. Sprinkle the crumbled bacon and asparagus mixture into the pie shells.

4. Sprinkle the cheese over the bacon and asparagus.

5. In a medium bowl, beat together the eggs, half-and-half, nutmeg, salt (if using), and pepper. Evenly pour the egg mixture on top of the cheese in both pie shells.

6. Bake the quiches until they are firm, 35 to 40 minutes. If the egg is darkening too much, cover with aluminum foil for the last 15 minutes. Let cool to room temperature before serving.

7. Store leftovers in a sealed container in the refrigerator for 3 days. They can also be wrapped tightly in plastic wrap and frozen for 2 to 3 months. Thaw and reheat in the oven.

TIP: To trim asparagus, pick up 5 to 8 stalks and hold at both ends of the vegetable. Bend the stem side until the end of the stalk easily snaps off. For this recipe, you can also leave 3 or 4 stalks whole for top decoration.

BREAKFAST BURRITOS

FREEZER-FRIENDLY, NUT-FREE, VEGETARIAN
YIELDS 6 BURRITOS

Think of this recipe as a template for whatever filling, make-ahead breakfast you crave. You can adjust any part of it based on what you have on hand. Serve these along with salsa, avocado, sour cream, and cilantro if desired.

3 tablespoons butter or extra-virgin olive oil, divided

6 eggs, beaten

1 cup canned black beans, drained and rinsed, or 1 cup Basic Black Beans (page 76)

1 bell pepper, diced

1 onion, diced

1 bunch scallions, green and white parts, chopped

6 flour tortillas

2 cups shredded Cheddar cheese

1. In a large nonstick skillet over medium-low heat, melt half of the butter.

2. Add the eggs and scramble until cooked through but not dry, stirring constantly so that the scrambled egg pieces are small. Remove them from the pan and set aside.

3. Add the remaining butter to the pan. Sauté the black beans, bell pepper, and onion until just softened, 2 to 3 minutes. Stir in the scallions.

4. One tortilla at a time, fill with ½ cup eggs, ¼ cup bean mixture, and ⅓ cup cheese. Carefully tuck in the ends and roll up the tortilla. Place burritos in a deep casserole dish.

5. Preheat the oven to low broil. Broil the burritos until slightly crispy and light brown. Remove from heat and allow to cool slightly before serving.

6. To freeze, wrap each burrito tightly in aluminum foil and place in a freezer-safe zip-top bag. Freeze for up to 3 months. To reheat, remove desired number of burritos and heat in a 350°F oven until cooked through.

PERFECT PITAS

FREEZER-FRIENDLY, DAIRY-FREE, NUT-FREE, VEGAN
YIELDS 8 PITAS

Store-bought pita bread is great, but it doesn't stand a chance against these made-from-scratch beauties. Soft and chewy, these super flavorful flatbreads can be used as mini pizza crusts, spread with your favorite topping, folded around fluffy scrambled eggs, or sliced into strips and dipped in soup or Black Bean Hummus (page 77).

1 packet yeast (about 2 teaspoons)
1 cup warm water
1 teaspoon granulated sugar

1 cup whole-wheat flour
1½ cups unbleached all-purpose flour, plus more for dusting and kneading

½ teaspoon salt (optional)
Extra-virgin olive oil

1. In a large bowl, combine the yeast with the warm water and sugar. Allow to sit until foamy, about 10 minutes.

2. Stir in the flours and salt (if using), and mix. Once the dough starts to come together, begin stirring with floured hands. If the dough feels sticky, add more flour, 1 teaspoon at a time. Transfer the dough to a floured surface and knead with your hands for about 5 minutes.

3. Drizzle the oil into the bowl you used to mix the dough and rub it up the sides. Return the dough to the bowl and loosely cover. Allow to rise for about 1½ hours, until doubled in size.

4. Divide the dough into 8 equal pieces. Using a rolling pin, roll each piece into a thin circle about 5 inches across.

5. Heat a large skillet over medium-low heat. Drizzle the skillet with olive oil and swirl to coat evenly. When oil is hot but not smoking, place one piece of flat dough in the skillet and cook until bubbles start to form, about 1 minute. Flip and cook on the other side for about 30 seconds. Repeat with remaining dough, adding more oil as needed.

6. Let cool slightly and serve.

7. Refrigerate in a container with a tightly fitting lid for up to 3 days. Or place cooked and cooled pitas in a freezer-safe container with parchment paper between each piece, and freeze for up to 3 months.

TIP: You can use a stand mixer with a dough hook attachment instead of kneading by hand.

PEANUT BUTTER BANANA SNACK BITES

FREEZER-FRIENDLY, DAIRY-FREE, GLUTEN-FREE, VEGAN
YIELDS 1 BANANA

Looking for quick, whole food snack ideas for your little one? This recipe is made from ingredients you probably have on hand already, and it's super easy to mix and match.

1 ripe banana

1 to 2 tablespoons creamy peanut butter

1 to 2 tablespoons toppings like crushed peanuts, mini chocolate chips, hemp hearts, ground flaxseed, and/or cinnamon

1. Peel the banana and cover the outside with a thin layer of peanut butter. Roll the entire banana in desired toppings until well covered. Cut the banana lengthwise and then slice it crosswise into bite-size pieces. Serve immediately.

2. Leftovers quickly become mushy in the refrigerator. Store leftovers in the freezer to toss into smoothies.

GREEN MACHINE BAKED FALAFEL

FREEZER-FRIENDLY, DAIRY-FREE, NUT-FREE, VEGAN
YIELDS ABOUT 14 FALAFEL BALLS

Like fritters, falafel is an easy-to-hold, veggie-packed meatless option perfect for any meal. Falafel balls are also portable, making them a great option for your next picnic in the park. And the edamame (shelled soybeans) add a bright green color and protein punch, while introducing soy, a common allergen.

2 (15-ounce) cans chickpeas, drained and rinsed

1 cup shelled edamame

¼ cup fresh herbs like cilantro, basil, parsley, and/or chives

1 onion, chopped

3 garlic cloves, peeled

1 tablespoon fresh lemon juice

½ teaspoon lemon zest

1 teaspoon cumin

Salt

Freshly ground black pepper

½ cup panko breadcrumbs

½ teaspoon baking powder

2 tablespoons extra-virgin olive oil

1. Preheat the oven to 375°F. Line a rimmed baking sheet with parchment paper.

2. In a food processor, combine the chickpeas, edamame, herbs, onion, garlic, lemon juice, lemon zest, cumin, salt, and pepper. Pulse until combined, leaving some large chunks of chickpeas.

3. Add the breadcrumbs and baking powder, and pulse until just combined.

4. Take about 2 tablespoons of chickpea mixture and form into a ball, then place on the prepared baking sheet. Repeat with remaining mixture, leaving space between each ball. Brush each ball with olive oil, covering all sides.

5. Bake until lightly browned, about 12 minutes.

6. Store leftover falafel balls in a sealed container in the refrigerator for up to 3 days. To freeze, cool to room temperature, place in a freezer bag, and freeze for up to 3 months.

EASY TZATZIKI SAUCE

GLUTEN-FREE, NUT-FREE, VEGETARIAN
YIELDS 2 CUPS

Toddlers love to dip, so we are always looking for ways to add nutritional value to meals through a tasty dip. This cool and creamy sauce is great for topping roasted veggies, dunking strips of Perfect Pitas (page 96), or serving alongside Green Machine Baked Falafel (page 99).

1 cup full-fat Greek yogurt

1 small cucumber, seeded and finely diced

¼ cup fresh herbs like dill, parsley, cilantro, and mint, chopped

2 tablespoons lemon juice

½ teaspoon lemon zest (optional)

Salt

Freshly ground black pepper

1. In a medium bowl, combine the yogurt with the cucumber, herbs, lemon juice, zest (if using), salt, and pepper. Mix well to incorporate.

2. Store leftovers in a sealed container in the refrigerator for up to 3 days.

BLUEBERRY LEMON SKILLET CAKE

NUT-FREE, VEGETARIAN
YIELDS 1 SKILLET CAKE

Ever had a Dutch baby? It's a giant oven-baked, puffed pancake, similar to a popover, and it is the inspiration for this recipe. It's so easy to make that this fluffy skillet cake might find its way onto your table at least once a week.

Butter for greasing the pan

1 cup milk

3 eggs

2 tablespoons granulated sugar (optional)

2 tablespoons fresh lemon juice

1 tablespoon lemon zest

½ teaspoon vanilla extract

½ cup unbleached all-purpose flour

2 cups blueberries, fresh or frozen

1. Preheat the oven to 325°F. Butter a 12-inch cast-iron or other ovenproof skillet.

2. In a medium bowl, whisk together the milk, eggs, sugar (if using), lemon juice, lemon zest, and vanilla extract. Stir in the flour.

3. Pour the mixture into the prepared skillet. Sprinkle the blueberries over the batter, and bake for about 35 minutes or until puffy and light brown around the edges. Serve warm.

4. Store leftovers in the refrigerator in a sealed container for up to 2 days.

TIP: Switch up this recipe by using chopped strawberries, blackberries, peaches, or pears—whatever's in season.

STRAWBERRY CHIA JAM

FREEZER-FRIENDLY, DAIRY-FREE, NUT-FREE, GLUTEN-FREE, VEGAN
YIELDS 2 CUPS

Making your own jam might sound a little intimidating, but with only three ingredients, why not give it a shot? This jam isn't as sweet as what you'll find in the grocery store, but it is a great way to add flavor to yogurt, oatmeal, and toast without adding a lot of sugar. Try it out on a baby-size PB&J. You may find yourself preferring this jam to sugary store-bought varieties, and your baby certainly won't know the difference!

4 cups fresh or frozen strawberries, hulled

1 tablespoon maple syrup or granulated sugar

¼ cup chia seeds

1. In a large saucepan over medium heat, cook the strawberries for about 10 minutes or until they start to break down.

2. Remove from heat and mash the strawberries with a fork until a sauce forms. Stir in the syrup or sugar.

3. Stir in the chia seeds and allow mixture to thicken and cool to room temperature. For a thicker consistency, stir in additional chia seeds 1 teaspoon at a time.

4. Transfer to a Mason jar with a tight-fitting lid and refrigerate. The jam will continue to thicken in the refrigerator.

5. Store in the refrigerator for up to 1 week, or freeze for up to 3 months and thaw in the refrigerator overnight before serving.

TIP: For a no-sugar-added, tart berry treat, omit the sugar.

CREAMY STRAWBERRY SMOOTHIE

FREEZER-FRIENDLY, DAIRY-FREE, GLUTEN-FREE, VEGAN
YIELDS ABOUT 1½ CUPS

This smoothie recipe was developed for families looking to boost calories in their baby's diet without using a sugary, dairy-based supplement. The texture is as creamy as strawberry ice cream, but you won't find any dairy in it. Split this smoothie with your babe; you'll love it, too!

6 large frozen strawberries
½ frozen banana
½ frozen avocado

1 cup full-fat coconut milk
¼ cup raw cashews

1. Put all the ingredients in a high-powered blender, and blend for about 1 minute, until smooth and creamy.

2. Freeze any leftover smoothie in an ice pop mold.

TIP: Full-fat coconut milk comes in a can and is often found in the international aisle of grocery stores. You can substitute any kind of milk in this recipe, or use soy yogurt for a creamier texture.

ROASTED STRAWBERRY PARFAITS

FREEZER-FRIENDLY, GLUTEN-FREE, NUT-FREE, VEGETARIAN
YIELDS 3 CUPS

Most flavored yogurt options in stores have quite a bit of added sugar. Sweetening your yogurt at home allows you to control the amount of sugar that goes in and also gives you the flexibility to flavor it any way you like. Here you'll roast strawberries, which brings out their intensely fruity flavor and softens them up nicely for baby.

2 cups fresh
strawberries, quartered

1 cup plain whole
milk yogurt

1. Preheat the oven to 375°F. Line a rimmed baking sheet with parchment paper.

2. Spread the strawberries in a single layer on the prepared baking sheet, and bake for 20 minutes.

3. Allow the berries to cool slightly, and then swirl them into the yogurt. Serve immediately or store in a sealed glass jar in the refrigerator for up to 2 to 3 days.

4. Roasted strawberries can be frozen separately from yogurt. Cool in the refrigerator and transfer to a freezer-safe container for up to 3 months.

TIP: Try adding roasted strawberries to a smoothie or an Open-Face PB and Unjelly Sandwich (page 108), or stir into oatmeal.

MINT CHOCOLATE CHIP ICE POPS

FREEZER-FRIENDLY, GLUTEN-FREE, NUT-FREE, VEGETARIAN
YIELDS ABOUT 6 SMALL POPSICLES

Peas in a pop? It's okay! Peas are a great source of plant-based protein for little ones, so these pops are great to have on hand for those days your child may not be very interested in eating. The peas, spinach, and mint make these treats a beautiful green color that looks just like the famous ice cream they're named after.

1½ cups full-fat vanilla Greek yogurt

¼ cup frozen peas

¼ cup frozen chopped spinach

¼ cup fresh mint leaves or ⅛ teaspoon spearmint extract

4 tablespoons mini chocolate chips

1. Combine the yogurt, peas, spinach, and mint leaves in a blender, and blend until smooth. Stir in the chocolate chips.

2. Pour or scoop the mixture into ice pop molds or paper cups and freeze until solid. (If using paper cups, see Banana-Avocado Teething Ice Pops on page 62 for the method.)

3. Store in the freezer for up to 3 months.

EASY PEANUT BUTTER PUDDING POPS

FREEZER-FRIENDLY, GLUTEN-FREE, VEGETARIAN
YIELDS 4 FROZEN POPS

The texture of these simple-to-make treats is reminiscent of the chocolate pudding pops of our childhoods. They're an excellent blend of protein and carbohydrates, making them the perfect snack for a hot summer day (and a great post-workout snack for parents).

2 very ripe bananas
1½ cups milk

½ cup creamy peanut butter
½ teaspoon vanilla extract

1. Combine all ingredients in a blender and blend until smooth and creamy.

2. Pour into ice pop molds and freeze until firm. The pudding pops will keep in the freezer for up to 3 months.

WHOLE FOOD OATMEAL COOKIE BARS

FREEZER-FRIENDLY, DAIRY-FREE, VEGAN
YIELDS ABOUT 12 BARS

Coming up with unprocessed homemade snacks that are as portable as store-bought options can be tricky, but here's a winner. These bars are incredibly simple, with only three main ingredients. The result is a soft, slightly chewy treat that tastes just like a freshly baked oatmeal cookie.

2 cups walnuts

1½ cups pitted dates

½ cup old-fashioned oats

1 tablespoon coconut oil, plus more if needed

1 teaspoon cinnamon

1. Line an 8-by-8-inch square pan with parchment paper.

2. In a food processor, combine all ingredients. Pulse until a crumbly paste or ball forms. Test to see if mixture sticks together when squeezed. If not, add more coconut oil 1 teaspoon at a time until mixture sticks together.

3. Transfer the mixture to the prepared pan, pressing in with fingers until evenly distributed. Chill in the refrigerator until firm, then slice into bars and wrap with plastic wrap.

4. Store in the refrigerator for best texture. Eat leftovers within 1 week. To freeze, individually wrap bars and store in a freezer-safe container for up to 3 months.

OPEN-FACE PB AND UNJELLY SANDWICH

DAIRY-FREE, VEGAN
YIELDS 2 OPEN-FACE SANDWICHES

So classic, yet unconventional. Once you introduce jelly to your little one, it's hard to un-know its wonders. For the under-one-year-old circuit, we start with a less sweet twist on this summer lunch staple. Baby-led weaning is all about serving whole, natural foods paired with family favorites for a nutritionally balanced meal, and that's exactly what this does.

1 tablespoon creamy peanut butter

2 slices whole-wheat bread, very lightly toasted

½ cup red seedless grapes, quartered

1. Spread a very thin layer (about ½ tablespoon) of creamy peanut butter onto each slice of bread.

2. Arrange the cut grapes on each slice of bread.

3. Cut each slice into 3 vertical strips, triangles, or whatever shape you desire. Serve immediately.

TIP: Team strawberry or grape? How about trying both? Or get creative by adding other juicy fruits, like halved or chopped blackberries or raspberries.

GOAT CHEESE–STUFFED SWEET POTATO WITH ROASTED GRAPES

GLUTEN-FREE, NUT-FREE, VEGETARIAN
YIELDS 4 BAKED SWEET POTATOES

Whether you're team marshmallow or team brown sugar and cinnamon on your sweet potatoes, let us introduce a new kid on the block: goat cheese and roasted grapes. You've gotta try it. It's a go-to when friends come over and you want to woo them with your fancy-schmancy cooking skills (shhh, it's actually so simple).

4 large sweet potatoes

2 cups halved red seedless grapes

1 teaspoon extra-virgin olive oil

Coarse salt

Freshly ground black pepper

4 ounces plain goat cheese

Pinch cinnamon (optional)

1. Preheat the oven to 375°F.

2. Pierce the potato skins with a fork. Wrap each tightly in aluminum foil. Bake for 45 to 60 minutes, or until potatoes are tender to the touch. Unwrap foil and cut a slit down the middle of each sweet potato. Cool for 5 to 10 minutes.

3. Increase oven temperature to 400°F.

4. Place the grapes on a nonstick baking sheet, drizzle with olive oil, and season with salt and pepper, tossing to coat. Roast for 10 to 15 minutes, or until the grapes begin to ooze jelly. Remove from the oven and let cool.

5. Stuff the sweet potatoes with goat cheese and grapes, then sprinkle with cinnamon (if using).

6. Refrigerate leftovers in a sealed container for up to 3 days.

TIP: For adults and kiddos over 1 year of age, you can add an extra pinch of coarse sea salt and a drizzle of honey for a decadent flavor enhancer.

SPAGHETTI SQUASH WITH MUSHROOM CREAM SAUCE

GLUTEN-FREE, NUT-FREE, VEGETARIAN
YIELDS 8 TO 10 CUPS

When this sauce is on the dinner menu, folks will know to get excited. This dish is warm and comforting and packed with savory veggies. Spaghetti squash provides a fun new texture for little ones to try and can be mixed and matched with any sauce.

1 spaghetti squash (about 2 pounds), halved and seeded

2 tablespoons extra-virgin olive oil

Coarse salt, to taste, divided

Freshly ground black pepper, to taste, divided

2 tablespoons butter

2 garlic cloves, minced, or 2 teaspoons minced

5 sage leaves, chopped, or ¼ teaspoon dried sage

8 ounces portobello mushrooms, sliced

1 cup heavy cream

¼ cup shredded Parmesan cheese (optional)

1. Preheat the oven to 400°F. Line a rimmed baking sheet with parchment paper.

2. On a large cutting board, carefully cut the squash in half lengthwise. Drizzle the insides of the squash with the olive oil and season with salt and pepper. Place cut-side down on the prepared baking sheet. Roast for about 1 hour or until squash is tender when pierced with a knife.

3. Meanwhile, in a medium skillet over medium-low heat, melt the butter. Add the garlic, sage, salt, pepper, and mushrooms and sauté for about 5 minutes or until mushrooms are tender.

4. Reduce heat to low and slowly pour in the heavy cream, stirring continuously. Cook on low until the sauce becomes smooth, about 10 minutes, then remove from heat.

5. When cool enough to handle, use a fork to gently scrape the squash to remove the flesh in long strands, and transfer to a medium bowl.

6. Portion out the spaghetti squash onto plates, and ladle the mushroom cream sauce on top. Garnish with cheese and salt.

7. Refrigerate leftovers in a container with a tightly fitting lid for up to 3 days.

TIP: Spaghetti squash is used in this recipe to replace traditional spaghetti noodles, but this sauce goes great with any type of pasta.

GREEN PEA AND SWEET CORN FRITTERS

FREEZER-FRIENDLY, DAIRY-FREE, NUT-FREE, VEGETARIAN
YIELDS ABOUT 12 SMALL FRITTERS

Fritters of all kinds are a baby-led weaning favorite. They are high in fat and calories and come in a convenient package perfect for little hands. Add to the list that you can make them ahead of time and that they are often loaded with veggies—we're sold.

1 cup thawed frozen peas, divided

1 cup fresh sweet corn cut from 2 ears, divided

3 eggs

2 scallions, chopped

2 garlic cloves, minced

1½ cups unbleached all-purpose flour

1 teaspoon baking powder

Fresh herbs such as basil, mint, parsley, or chives (optional)

Salt

Freshly ground black pepper

¼ cup extra-virgin olive oil, divided

1. Add ½ cup peas, ½ cup corn, eggs, scallions, and garlic to a food processor, and pulse until well combined. Add the flour, baking powder, fresh herbs (if using), salt, and pepper. Pulse again until combined.

2. Scoop the mixture into a medium bowl and fold in the remaining peas and corn.

3. Heat 2 tablespoons olive oil in a skillet over medium heat. Form the fritter mixture into patties 2 tablespoons at a time. Fry the fritters in batches for 2 to 3 minutes on each side, or until golden brown, adding more oil as needed.

4. Store leftovers in a sealed container in the refrigerator for 2 to 3 days, or in the freezer for up to 3 months. Thaw, then heat in a skillet 1 or 2 at a time for a quick meal.

GARLICKY SAUTÉED WHITE BEANS

DAIRY-FREE, GLUTEN-FREE, NUT-FREE
YIELDS 4½ CUPS

These flavorful beans are versatile and packed with nutrients. Make these ahead of time and serve them with any meal—spoon over sautéed spinach or baby kale, mash and spread on toast, or serve with fruit for a quick and easy lunch.

¼ cup extra-virgin olive oil

4 garlic cloves, minced

¼ to ½ cup low-sodium chicken or vegetable broth, divided

2 (15.5-ounce) cans cannellini beans

1 (28-ounce) can low-sodium diced tomatoes

2 tablespoons minced fresh herbs such as sage, thyme, parsley, and/or rosemary

Salt

Freshly ground black pepper

1. In a large skillet over medium heat, heat the olive oil. Add the garlic and cook until fragrant, about 2 minutes. Whisk in ¼ cup of broth and cook for 2 more minutes.

2. Add the beans and tomatoes, bring to a simmer, and cook for 15 to 20 minutes. If the beans begin to look dry, add more broth as needed while simmering.

3. Season with fresh herbs, salt, and pepper.

4. Store leftovers in a sealed container in the refrigerator for up to 3 days.

ONE-PAN LENTIL DAL

DAIRY-FREE, GLUTEN-FREE, NUT-FREE, VEGAN
YIELDS 6 CUPS

This is a favorite recipe for getting dinner on the table in less than 30 minutes. And it only uses one pan! We are sometimes still surprised by how well our toddlers love iron-rich dishes like this dal, which many would not consider "toddler" food. For an even faster cook time, soak lentils for 2 to 3 hours prior to cooking.

2 tablespoons coconut oil

1 onion, diced

2 large carrots, diced

4 garlic cloves, minced

1 tablespoon finely chopped ginger root

1 teaspoon curry powder

½ teaspoon cumin

¼ teaspoon salt

1 (28-ounce) can low-sodium diced tomatoes

1 cup low-sodium vegetable broth or water

1 can full-fat coconut milk

1 cup red lentils, rinsed

1. In a large skillet over medium heat, melt the coconut oil. Add the onion, carrots, garlic, and ginger. Cook until vegetables start to soften. Stir in the curry powder, cumin, and salt, and cook for 1 to 2 minutes more.

2. Pour in the tomatoes, broth, and coconut milk, then add the lentils. Bring to a simmer, stirring occasionally. Cover and reduce heat to medium-low. Cook, still stirring occasionally, until lentils are tender, about 20 minutes. Serve warm.

3. Refrigerate leftovers in an airtight container for up to 3 days, or freeze for up to 2 months.

TIP: Substitute ½ teaspoon ground ginger for fresh ginger.

SAUTÉED VEGGIE PITA PIZZAS WITH QUICK KALE PESTO

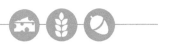

GLUTEN-FREE, VEGETARIAN
YIELDS 2 (5- TO 6-INCH) PIZZAS, 1 CUP PESTO

There is something so summery about the taste of pesto. One taste of it takes you to early June and an herb garden that is bursting with new green leaves and colorful blooms. This version could not be simpler to whip up and takes homemade pizza to the next level. Serve this pizza cut into strips or larger slices to allow your baby to practice taking different-size bites.

For the pesto

3 cups baby kale or spinach

1 cup fresh basil leaves

½ cup grated Parmesan cheese

½ cup almonds, walnuts, or pine nuts

5 garlic cloves, peeled

¼ to ½ cup extra-virgin olive oil, plus 1 tablespoon, divided

For the pizzas

2 tablespoons extra-virgin olive oil

1 small zucchini, thinly sliced

2 pitas, homemade (see page 96) or store-bought

¼ cup homemade kale pesto

1 pint cherry tomatoes, quartered

1 (8-ounce) ball fresh mozzarella cheese, thinly sliced or torn into small chunks

To make the pesto

1. Combine the kale, basil, Parmesan cheese, nuts, garlic, and olive oil in a food processor.

2. Pulse until the desired texture is reached. Set aside.

To make the pizzas

3. In a medium skillet over medium heat, heat the olive oil. Add the zucchini and lightly sauté for 2 to 3 minutes.

4. Preheat the broiler on low.

5. Spread the pitas with pesto and top with zucchini, cherry tomatoes, and mozzarella. Place on a baking sheet and broil for about 5 minutes, until cheese bubbles and lightly browns. Serve warm.

6. Store leftovers in the refrigerator in a sealed container for up to 3 days. You will not use all the pesto, so to freeze leftovers, pour into an ice cube tray and freeze until solid, then pop out into a freezer bag. Freeze for up to 6 months.

TIP: Try leftover pesto as a spread for toast or mixed with a little mayo as a dip for sweet potato fries.

VEGGIE LASAGNA

FREEZER-FRIENDLY, NUT-FREE, VEGETARIAN
YIELDS 1 (9-BY-13-INCH) LASAGNA

You won't miss the meat in this lasagna. This rich, colorful dish has been a staple holiday main course in Ellen's home for years, featuring rich red tomato sauce, vibrant green spinach, and colorful shredded carrots layered between pasta and savory cheeses. This is a great make-ahead meal to prepare in batches and freeze for a quick dinner.

6 to 9 lasagna noodles (whole wheat or regular)

Extra-virgin olive oil, for greasing the pan

1 (10-ounce) box frozen spinach, thawed and well-drained

1½ cups grated carrots (5 or 6 medium carrots)

1 (15-ounce) container whole milk ricotta cheese

½ cup shaved or shredded Parmesan cheese

1 cup diced onion

1 cup chopped bell pepper

1 tablespoon Italian seasoning

1 tablespoon minced garlic

2 teaspoons salt

1 teaspoon freshly ground black pepper

1 (26-ounce) jar low-sodium marinara sauce

3 cups shredded mozzarella cheese, divided

1. In a large stockpot, bring 8 cups of water to a boil. Add the lasagna noodles, and cook until al dente. Drain, rinse noodles with cold water, and set aside.

2. Preheat the oven to 350°F. Lightly grease a 9-by-13-inch casserole dish with olive oil.

3. In a medium bowl, combine the spinach, carrots, ricotta cheese, Parmesan cheese, onion, bell pepper, Italian seasoning, garlic, salt, and pepper. Mix until all ingredients are thoroughly incorporated.

4. Spread ½ cup marinara sauce in the bottom of the prepared casserole dish.

5. Cover the sauce with a layer of lasagna noodles. Layer with half of the ricotta mix, 1 cup mozzarella cheese, and ½ cup marinara sauce. Repeat layering, and top with the remaining cup of mozzarella cheese.

6. Bake uncovered 40 to 45 minutes, until bubbly and the top layer of cheese is browned. Let the lasagna set 15 to 20 minutes before serving.

7. Refrigerate leftovers in a container with a tightly fitting lid for up to 3 days. Uncooked lasagna can be wrapped tightly in plastic wrap and frozen for up to 3 months. To prepare, thaw in refrigerator overnight and bake according to recipe directions.

TIP: If your family is full of meat lovers, then absolutely add browned ground beef into the marinara sauce for an additional punch of iron.

LIZZIE'S HOMEMADE CHICKEN POT PIE

NUT-FREE

YIELDS 2 (9-INCH) PIES OR 1 (9-BY-13-INCH) CASSEROLE

"No more meatloaf, no more steak; it's chicken soup that you have to bake. It's made with veggies, it's made with love, a pinch of spices, and other stuff. It's not for momma, it's not for me, it's for our little Ruth Marie." Yes, Ellen and her husband actually wrote a song for their daughter about this chicken pot pie recipe. Because it is *that* good. Clearly a family favorite—so much so that it was requested by name as the entrée choice for Ruth's second birthday.

For the pie crust

1½ cups unbleached all-purpose flour

1 stick chilled butter, cut into cubes

¼ cup ice cold water

For the pot pie

6 tablespoons butter

1 onion, diced

⅔ cup unbleached all-purpose flour

½ teaspoon salt

½ teaspoon freshly ground black pepper

3 cups low-sodium chicken broth

1⅓ cups milk

3 cups shredded cooked chicken (see Tip)

3 (12-ounce) bags frozen mixed vegetables, or 3 white potatoes, peeled and diced

½ teaspoon fresh or dried parsley, plus more for garnish if desired

½ teaspoon sage

½ teaspoon rosemary, plus more for garnish if desired

½ teaspoon thyme

1 egg white, lightly beaten (optional)

To make the crust

1. In a large bowl, add the flour. Pressing with the back of a fork, cut the butter into the flour until the dough becomes pea-sized chunks. Add the water a little at a time, continuing to work the flour, until it becomes a solid mass. Do not overstir.

2. Turn the dough onto a square of waxed paper, top with another piece of waxed paper, and roll with rolling pin. Press the dough into the bottom and sides of a 9-by-13-inch baking pan, and carefully cut around the top edges of the pan. Use the extra dough strips to decorate the top.

To make the pot pies

1. Preheat the oven to 375°F. In a medium saucepan over medium heat, melt the butter. Add the onion and cook, stirring occasionally for 2 minutes or until tender.

2. Add the flour, salt, and pepper. Then stir in the broth and milk, cooking and stirring until bubbly and thickened.

3. Add the shredded chicken and mixed vegetables or potatoes, mixing well.

4. Add the parsley, sage, rosemary, and thyme, then remove from heat.

5. Spoon the hot mixture into the crust-lined baking pan. Decorate with leftover strips of dough. Brush the dough with the egg white (if using), then garnish with additional fresh or dried herbs, if desired.

6. Bake for 30 to 40 minutes, or until the crust is golden brown. Serve warm.

7. Refrigerate in a sealed container for up to 3 days, or cool, wrap tightly, and freeze for a later meal. Thaw overnight and bake to reheat.

TIP: You can get your chicken from a whole 3- to 4-pound chicken, boiled and shredded, or 5 to 6 chicken breasts boiled. Reserve the water from the boiled chicken for the broth.

CHICKEN DIVINE

FREEZER-FRIENDLY, GLUTEN-FREE, NUT-FREE
YIELDS 16 TO 18 CUPS, INCLUDING RICE

A perfectly named recipe, this family dish is a rich, creamy, drip-down-your-chin family favorite. It also has all the components of a balanced, energy-filled plate for your baby (and your whole family)!

1 stick butter, plus more for greasing the pan

4 tablespoons unbleached all-purpose flour

2 cups low-sodium chicken broth

2 cups milk

2 cups mayonnaise

1 cup water

1 tablespoon curry powder

2 teaspoons lemon juice

4 cups chopped cooked broccoli (2 medium heads broccoli)

3 cups shredded cooked chicken

8 ounces shredded sharp Cheddar cheese

3 to 4 cups cooked brown rice

1. Preheat the oven to 375°F. Lightly grease a 9-by-13-inch baking pan.

2. In a medium saucepan over medium-low heat, melt the butter. Add the flour and whisk until smooth and bubbly.

3. Slowly whisk in the chicken broth and milk. Bring to a gentle boil and cook, whisking constantly, until the soup thickens, about 5 to 7 minutes.

4. Stir in the mayonnaise, water, curry powder, and lemon juice, bring to a boil over low heat, and cook for 3 to 4 minutes.

5. In the baking pan, mix the broccoli and shredded chicken. Pour the sauce on top. Sprinkle with the cheese. Bake for 20 to 25 minutes or until bubbly.

6. Serve atop a warm bed of rice. Refrigerate leftovers in a sealed container for up to 3 days, or freeze for up to 3 months.

EASY TUNA QUESADILLA

NUT-FREE

YIELDS 2 QUESADILLAS

Here's a nontraditional twist on a classic tuna melt, perfect for an easy last-minute lunch. This dish includes three allergens, so try this recipe after you've confirmed your baby's tolerance for fish, dairy, and wheat.

1 (2.6-ounce) pouch chunk light tuna in water

¼ cup plain Greek yogurt

¼ cup shredded Cheddar cheese

1 teaspoon lemon juice

Pinch cumin (optional)

Pinch garlic powder (optional)

2 (8- to 10-inch) whole-wheat tortillas

1 tablespoon butter

1. In a small bowl, combine the tuna, yogurt, cheese, lemon juice, and cumin and garlic (if using). Divide the filling mixture evenly between two tortillas, smoothing to cover entire surface to edges. Fold the tortillas in half.

2. Heat a cast-iron skillet on medium heat, add butter, and swirl the pan to coat. Place the filled tortillas in the skillet and cook until desired brownness. Carefully flip over quesadillas with a small spatula, and cook on the other side.

3. Let cool before serving. Cut quesadilla in half or quarters for easy serving for little hands.

4. These quesadillas should be eaten immediately. Store any leftovers in the refrigerator for no more than 2 days, and for best quality, reheat them in the oven.

TIP: Serve these quesadillas with a side of Basic Black Beans (page 76) and sliced avocado, and garnish with diced tomatoes. Or throw these ingredients into the quesadillas before cooking.

SIMPLE SHRIMP FAJITAS

FREEZER-FRIENDLY, DAIRY-FREE, NUT-FREE
YIELDS 10 TO 12 FAJITAS

When serving notoriously hard-to-eat-without-making-a-mess foods like fajitas or tacos to babies and toddlers, we like to offer deconstructed versions. This keeps up our mission of "one family, one meal" while making sure our children are able to handle their self-feeding duties without frustration. Serve a few pieces of shrimp and veggies with whole or quartered tortillas and sour cream and salsa for dipping.

1 pound fresh or thawed frozen shrimp, peeled, deveined, and butterflied

1 teaspoon chili powder

1 teaspoon garlic powder

1 teaspoon cumin

2 tablespoons extra-virgin olive oil, divided

1 bell pepper, sliced into thin strips

1 onion, sliced into thin strips

1 zucchini, cut into thin strips

10 to 12 soft flour or corn tortillas

Sour cream, salsa, avocado, and cilantro, for serving (optional)

1. In a large bowl, combine the shrimp, chili powder, garlic powder, and cumin, and toss to coat. Set aside.

2. Heat 1 tablespoon of olive oil in a large skillet over medium-high heat. Add the bell pepper, onion, and zucchini, and sauté until softened. Remove from heat.

3. Add remaining 1 tablespoon olive oil to skillet. Add shrimp and cook until no longer pink, about 5 to 7 minutes. Return cooked vegetables to the pan with the shrimp.

4. To serve, top a tortilla with warm shrimp and vegetables, or offer a deconstructed fajita. Add optional toppings (if using).

5. Refrigerate leftovers in a sealed container for up to 3 days.

TIP: Quickly and safely thaw frozen shrimp by placing in a colander under cold running water.

CREAMY POLENTA BOLOGNESE

NUT-FREE

YIELDS 3 CUPS POLENTA, 4 CUPS BOLOGNESE

This hearty dinner offers a unique take on classic spaghetti and meat sauce. Polenta is a great baby-led weaning food, thanks to its soft, creamy texture. When chilled, polenta can also be cut into easy-to-grasp-patties and pan-fried—delicious served alongside scrambled eggs in the morning.

For the polenta

3 cups low-sodium chicken or vegetable broth, or water

½ cup whole-grain cornmeal

2 tablespoons butter

¼ cup shredded Parmesan cheese

For the Bolognese

1 tablespoon extra-virgin olive oil

1 large onion, diced

4 garlic cloves, minced

2 large carrots, diced

1 pound ground beef

1 (28-ounce) can low-sodium diced tomatoes

2 tablespoons chopped fresh basil

Salt

Freshly ground black pepper

To make the polenta

1. In a medium saucepan over high heat, bring the broth to a boil.

2. Add the cornmeal, whisking constantly to prevent clumps from forming. Reduce heat to medium-low and continue cooking for about 20 minutes, stirring occasionally as the mixture thickens. Be careful—bubbling polenta can splatter and cause burns!

3. Taste for doneness; most of the gritty texture should be gone, yielding a creamy result.

4. Remove the pot from the heat, and stir in the butter and cheese.

To make the Bolognese

1. In a large skillet over medium heat, heat the olive oil. Add the onion, garlic, and carrots, and cook until very soft.

2. Increase heat to medium-high and add the ground beef, breaking up large chunks. Cook for 10 to 12 minutes or until beef is cooked through and no pink remains.

3. Reduce heat to medium-low and add the tomatoes and basil. Cook until the sauce thickens, 20 to 30 minutes. Season with salt and pepper.

4. Serve the sauce over warm polenta.

5. Store leftovers in a sealed container in the refrigerator for 2 days. Freeze leftover sauce in a freezer-safe container for up to 3 months.

TIP: Polenta can be served as runny or thick as you prefer. Look for precooked polenta cornmeal for quicker cooking times.

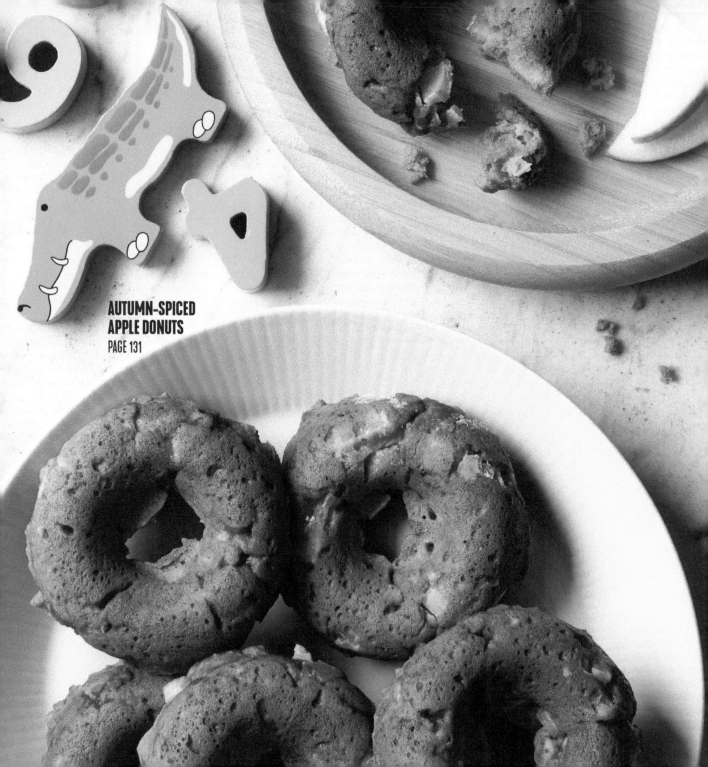

**AUTUMN-SPICED
APPLE DONUTS**
PAGE 131

12 MONTHS AND BEYOND AT THE FAMILY TABLE

WHAT TO EXPECT

Happy birthday, baby! The goal for this age and going forward is to continue to foster a confident, adventurous eater who is regularly consuming a variety of meats, grains, fruits, vegetables, and dairy prepared in different combinations of textures, flavors, and spices. Babies are still very accepting of new foods at this time, but watch out—strong food preferences will soon emerge. Be careful not to start relying on too much processed and convenient "kid foods." Continued exposure to healthy whole ingredients is essential to avoid the slippery slope into unhealthy food expectations.

As your baby becomes more mobile, their appetite may also increase. Watch for hunger cues to see if a mid-morning or afternoon snack is needed. Appetites can also fluctuate greatly during this time, especially during hard teething weeks. Previously favorite foods may get thrown onto the floor, but it won't last long. Cyclic preferences are common at this age—they come and go.

Baby's Motor Skills

As your baby builds motor skills, you can help their progress. Continue to encourage the use of self-feeding with utensils, perhaps transitioning from soft-tipped self-feeders to miniature, blunt-edged, stainless steel forks and spoons. Let your child practice with dipping and using a spoon in thinner liquids and soups.

Your child's first birthday is a great opportunity to introduce an open cup. Spills happen, and this skill set is something that takes time. Keep in mind, of course, that smaller pours equal smaller spills. Use both open cups and straws, as each method helps develop different mouth muscles.

Eating at This Stage

If you haven't done so yet, now is a great time to begin a schedule for meals and snacks. This schedule can be flexible, but having planned mealtimes and snack times is a great way to avoid the toddler trap of grazing throughout the day. A schedule also ensures you always have an answer to the question, "Can I have a snack?" The answer may be, "Yes, snack time will be right after your bath."

A sample schedule might look like this: breakfast 8:00 a.m. (within 30 minutes to an hour of waking if appetite is there), snack 10:00 a.m., lunch 12:00 p.m., snack 2:30 p.m., dinner 5:00 p.m.

You may choose to begin offering meals family-style, allowing toddlers to choose how much and which foods they would like to try. This method allows toddlers to choose their own portion size (with some assistance) and supports their ability to eat the amount they need.

Every child is different. By the end of the day, some young toddlers are not very interested in eating. On the other hand, you may find some early risers aren't hungry right away. Both are totally normal. You will discover your babe's schedule and find what meals they are most interested in, and you can simply optimize nutrition at those times.

Introducing Cow's Milk

Here are some tips based on questions we frequently receive about introducing cow's milk:

CONTINUE BREASTFEEDING AS LONG AS YOU AND YOUR BABY WOULD LIKE. Breast milk has more fat and nutrients than cow's milk and is the ideal choice as long as you and your baby are up for it. If you choose to continue breastfeeding, your baby's nutrient needs are covered and you don't have to introduce cow's milk (unless you would like to).

GO WITH WHOLE MILK. If you're weaning from breast milk or formula, you can offer whole cow's milk (3.25 percent fat) to provide key nutrients as part of meals and snacks.

SUPPLEMENT NECESSARY NUTRIENTS. If you're not offering whole cow's milk regularly, offer foods rich in calcium, fat, and calories often. Continue supplementing with vitamin D drops. Cow's milk is not an absolutely necessary part of a healthy diet as long as these nutrients are provided by food.

DON'T RELY ON PLANT-BASED MILK YET. Plant-based milks (especially almond, coconut, and rice milk) are usually too low in protein, fat, and calories to be appropriate as a daily beverage for toddlers. But they can still be used in cooking or smoothies. Soy milk is the best option if offering plant-based milk to toddlers under age 2.

SERVE MILK WITH FOOD. Offer milk in an open cup as part of a meal or snack (rather than offering milk in between meal or snack time). Limit to 16 ounces per day.

Recipes at This Stage

With pincer grasp in full force, your baby is becoming more adept. That means you can switch up the sizes and shapes of the foods you offer in whatever way works best for your family. Many toddlers do well with small pieces, or you can simply begin to provide food for your infant in the same way that you present it to the rest of the family (keeping in mind the safety guidelines on page 17).

A note on added sugars: Some families choose to completely avoid added sugars (this include granulated sugar, brown sugar, molasses, cane sugar, maple syrup, honey, agave, coconut sugar, and brown rice syrup) well into toddlerhood. While this is a great goal—sugar is definitely not a necessary part of a toddler's diet—we are a little more laid-back about this ingredient. Because of our focus on developing a healthy lifelong relationship with food, we want to avoid putting extra pressure on parents to completely rule out sugars, especially as part of a whole food, healthy lifestyle. Some of the recipes in this section contain added sugars. Feel free to omit the sugar in any of the recipes as you see fit.

Many of the recipes in this chapter are more complex and contain many ingredients you wouldn't necessarily picture at the kids' buffet. But that's the point. Early exposure to every kind of food is how adventurous eaters are created. When you start reading the recipes for dishes like Pappy's Chili (page 163) and Mexican Chicken Casserole (page 165), just remember that they are all a part of the exposure that will help your baby broaden their culinary interests. Basically, this group of recipes is full of family favorites that we are sure you will enjoy for years to come.

AUTUMN-SPICED APPLE DONUTS

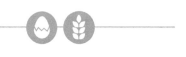

FREEZER-FRIENDLY, DAIRY-FREE, NUT-FREE, VEGETARIAN
YIELDS 12 DONUTS

Each fall, the orchards around our part of the country feature the most delicious apple cider donuts. Luckily, you don't have to wait for fall to try this easy-to-whip-up donut recipe.

Oil or butter, for greasing

1 cup unbleached, all-purpose flour

1 cup oat flour (see Tip)

1 teaspoon baking soda

1 teaspoon pumpkin pie spice

1 teaspoon cinnamon

½ teaspoon salt

½ teaspoon ground ginger

½ cup coconut oil

¼ cup brown sugar

2 eggs

1 teaspoon vanilla extract

1 cup applesauce or pear sauce

1 cup peeled, cored, and finely chopped apples or pears

1. Preheat the oven to 350°F. Lightly grease a donut or muffin tin.

2. In a bowl, combine the flours, baking soda, pumpkin pie spice, cinnamon, salt, and ginger, and whisk to combine. Set aside.

3. In the bowl of a stand mixer, mix the coconut oil and brown sugar until light and airy. Add the eggs and vanilla extract and whisk again. Stir in the applesauce or pear sauce and chopped fruit.

4. Stir the dry ingredients into the wet ingredients until incorporated. Pour the batter into the donut or muffin tin. Bake 25 to 30 minutes or until golden brown and springy to the touch.

5. Store in a tightly sealed container in the refrigerator for up to 3 days. Freeze in a freezer-safe container for up to 3 months.

CHOCOLATE DONUT HOLES

FREEZER-FRIENDLY, DAIRY-FREE, GLUTEN-FREE, VEGAN
YIELDS 24 DONUT HOLES

Getting young toddlers involved in the kitchen is a great sensory activity and also a way to increase their interest in trying new foods. For simple recipes like this one, little hands are helpful in shaping the mixture into perfectly imperfect balls.

1 cup pitted dates
1 cup old-fashioned oats
½ cup almonds

½ cup unsweetened shredded coconut
3 tablespoons coconut oil, plus more as needed

2 tablespoons unsweetened cocoa powder
1 teaspoon vanilla extract

1. Line a baking sheet with parchment paper.

2. Put all the ingredients in a food processor and pulse until well combined. Squeeze to see that it sticks together. If the mixture is still crumbly, add in more coconut oil, 1 teaspoon at a time.

3. Roll the mixture into balls and place on the prepared baking sheet. Refrigerate until firm. Remove from the pan and serve.

4. Refrigerate leftovers in a container with a tightly fitting lid for up to 1 week. Store in a freezer-safe container for up to 3 months.

TIP: These donut holes are portable and do not require refrigeration if you're only storing them for a couple of days. They can be stored in the refrigerator to keep the mixture firm and last longer.

CHOCOLATE ALMOND BREAKFAST BITES

FREEZER-FRIENDLY, VEGETARIAN
YIELDS 24 COOKIES

Cookies for breakfast is a concept we are all about, especially on busy workday or school day mornings when you just need to grab something on the way out the door. Including a breakfast cookie recipe in your meal prep routine can be a yummy lifesaver or a quick addition to breakfast or snack time.

2 cups old-fashioned oats

1 cup unbleached all-purpose flour

⅓ cup ground flaxseed

2 tablespoons brown sugar

½ teaspoon baking powder

½ teaspoon baking soda

¼ teaspoon salt

2 ripe bananas, mashed

1 egg, lightly beaten

2½ tablespoons coconut oil, melted and cooled to room temperature

2½ tablespoons butter, melted and cooled to room temperature

3 tablespoons milk

2 teaspoons vanilla extract

½ cup toasted sliced almonds, finely chopped

½ cup mini chocolate chips or cacao nibs

1. Preheat the oven to 350°F. Line a baking sheet with parchment paper.

2. In a large bowl, mix together the oats, flour, flaxseed, brown sugar, baking powder, baking soda, and salt.

3. In a medium bowl, mix together the bananas, egg, coconut oil, butter, milk, and vanilla extract. Add the wet ingredients to the dry and combine without overmixing. Fold in the almonds and chocolate.

4. Drop by spoonfuls onto the prepared baking sheet. Bake for 12 to 15 minutes.

5. These can be stored on the countertop in a sealed container or in a reusable zip-top bag for up to 1 week. You can also freeze the dough (separated into spoonfuls), for up to 3 months, baking batches as needed (no need to thaw).

BUTTERNUT SQWAFFLES

FREEZER-FRIENDLY, NUT-FREE, VEGETARIAN
YIELDS 3½ CUPS BATTER

"Sqwaffles? What are those?" you might ask. Well, it turns out that squash makes a great add-in to waffle batter. And waffles are baby-led weaning favorites thanks to their versatility and easy-to-grab shape. This recipe combines nutrient-packed butternut squash with warm spices. Try spreading them with Greek yogurt and Strawberry Chia Jam (page 102).

2 to 3 tablespoons extra-virgin olive oil for greasing the waffle iron

1 cup unbleached all-purpose flour

½ cup old-fashioned oats

2 teaspoons baking powder

1 teaspoon baking soda

1 teaspoon cinnamon

¼ teaspoon nutmeg

¼ teaspoon cloves

2 eggs

1¼ cups milk

1 cup cooked butternut squash, mashed or puréed

1 teaspoon vanilla extract

1. Oil and preheat a waffle iron.

2. In a large bowl, mix together the flour, oats, baking powder, baking soda, cinnamon, nutmeg, and cloves.

3. In a medium bowl, mix together the eggs, milk, butternut squash, and vanilla extract.

4. Pour the wet ingredients into dry, and stir until just combined.

5. Pour ¼ cup of batter onto the hot waffle iron and cook until steaming stops, about 4 minutes. Repeat with remaining batter. Serve immediately, or store.

6. Refrigerate cooked waffles in a sealed container for up to 3 days, or freeze for up to 3 months. Just pop them in a toaster oven to reheat.

WAFFLE SANDWICHES

NUT-FREE, VEGETARIAN
YIELDS 1 WAFFLE

This is a great recovery dish to make after a morning at the gym. It delivers protein, healthy fats, complex carbohydrates, and delicious tastes. As for baby, cut it into little pincer-grasp pieces—it's like a bento box scramble!

5 or 6 cherry tomatoes, quartered

1 tablespoon balsamic vinegar

1 teaspoon extra-virgin olive oil

1 teaspoon minced garlic

¼ teaspoon salt, plus more for garnish (optional)

¼ teaspoon freshly ground black pepper, plus more for garnish (optional)

1 Butternut Sqwaffle (page 134) or any frozen waffle

1 teaspoon butter

1 egg

1 tablespoon plain goat cheese, crumbled

¼ avocado, sliced

Grated Parmesan cheese for garnish (optional)

1. Preheat the broiler.

2. Place the cherry tomato segments in a small, foil-lined baking pan. Toss with the balsamic vinegar, olive oil, minced garlic, salt, and pepper (if using). Broil for 5 to 7 minutes.

3. Toast the sqwaffle in a toaster or on the bottom rack of your oven while the tomato mixture is cooking.

4. In a small skillet over medium-high heat, melt the butter. Fry or scramble the egg. Slide onto the sqwaffle. Top the egg with crumbled goat cheese and avocado slices. Garnish with salt, pepper, and Parmesan cheese (if using). Serve immediately.

SIMPLE ONE-PAN SHAKSHUKA (BAKED EGGS)

FREEZER-FRIENDLY, DAIRY-FREE, NUT-FREE, VEGETARIAN
YIELDS 6 CUPS

This awesome recipe, a traditional meal in North African countries and the Middle East, is great for those days when dinnertime sneaks up way too quickly. It's made with ingredients you probably have on hand already and comes together in less than 30 minutes. Serve with Perfect Pitas (page 96) or any store-bought flatbread.

1 tablespoon extra-virgin olive oil

2 garlic cloves, minced

1 onion, diced

1 bell pepper, diced

1 teaspoon paprika

1 (28-ounce) can low-sodium diced tomatoes

4 eggs

1. In a large cast-iron skillet over medium heat, heat the olive oil.

2. Add the garlic, onion, and bell pepper. Cook for about 3 minutes, or until the mixture becomes fragrant and the onions begin to soften. Sprinkle with paprika and cook for about 2 minutes more.

3. Pour in the tomatoes and bring to a simmer. Crack eggs into a small bowl one at a time and slide into the sauce. Cover and let simmer until yolks are firm.

TIP: To serve, scoop an egg and some of the rich tomato sauce onto your baby's plate, slicing the egg into strips for easy gripping and dipping.

FLOURLESS CASHEW BUTTER BLENDER MUFFINS

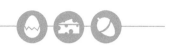

FREEZER-FRIENDLY, DAIRY-FREE, GLUTEN-FREE, VEGETARIAN
YIELDS 12 MUFFINS

There are few things handier than a good go-to muffin recipe for your family. This nutty, lightly sweet muffin is a great high-calorie and nutrient-dense version of a classic kid fave.

Cooking spray, for greasing

1 cup smooth cashew butter (you can also use almond, peanut, or sunflower seed butter)

½ cup mashed cooked sweet potato

½ cup mashed ripe banana

3 eggs

4 tablespoons maple syrup

1 teaspoon vanilla extract

½ teaspoon baking soda

½ teaspoon ground ginger

½ teaspoon cinnamon

1. Preheat the oven to 350°F. Grease a 12-cup muffin tin with cooking spray (or use paper muffin liners).

2. Add all the ingredients to a high-powered blender or food processor, and pulse until smooth. Pour the mixture into the prepared muffin tin, leaving 1 inch at the top of each muffin cup.

3. Bake for 15 to 20 minutes or until a toothpick inserted into the center comes out clean.

4. Store leftovers in a sealed container in the refrigerator for up to 1 week, or freeze in a freezer-safe container for up to 3 months.

PEANUT BUTTER BANANA FRENCH TOAST STICKS

VEGETARIAN
YIELDS 4 TO 5 STICKS

French toast is typically a leisurely weekend breakfast, but it's really pretty quick to throw together, even on busy mornings. The banana in this recipe adds sweetness, while the peanut butter packs in calories, protein, and healthy fats.

1 ripe banana, mashed
1 egg
¼ cup milk

1 tablespoon creamy peanut butter
1 teaspoon vanilla extract

1 tablespoon butter or coconut oil
2 pieces bread, sliced into sticks

1. In a bowl, add the mashed banana, egg, milk, peanut butter, and vanilla extract, and mix until well combined.

2. In a cast-iron skillet over medium heat, melt the butter or coconut oil, swirling to coat the bottom of the pan evenly.

3. Dip the bread sticks into the banana-egg mixture and coat evenly. Add to the hot pan and cook for about 2 minutes on each side, until the egg mixture cooks through and is lightly browned. Serve warm.

4. Store leftovers in a sealed container in the refrigerator for up to 3 days.

BLACK CHERRY BAKED OATMEAL

NUT-FREE, VEGETARIAN
YIELDS 4 TO 6 SERVINGS

Baked oatmeal might sound odd, but this recipe is full of protein and great on a cold morning. Think of this as a coffee cake that's gone to nutritional school! The flaxseed and oatmeal both add essential fiber and nutrients, while the black cherries add color, flavor, and antioxidants.

Butter or extra-virgin olive oil for greasing the pan

2 cups fresh black cherries, chopped

2 cups old-fashioned oats

1½ cups milk

1 cup plain yogurt

2 eggs, lightly beaten

¼ cup ground flaxseed

¼ cup granulated sugar (optional)

1 teaspoon vanilla extract

½ teaspoon baking powder

¼ teaspoon baking soda

½ teaspoon salt

1. Preheat the oven to 350°F. Grease a 9-by-9-inch square baking dish.

2. Place all the ingredients in a large bowl, and stir until well combined.

3. Transfer to the prepared baking dish and bake for 25 minutes, or until oats are fully cooked.

4. Let cool slightly, and cut into squares to serve.

ZUCCHINI OAT COOKIES

FREEZER-FRIENDLY, NUT-FREE, VEGETARIAN
YIELDS ABOUT 20 COOKIES

Chewy and subtly sweet, these hidden-veggie cookies have been a favorite of our kids since they were babies. While we aren't huge fans of sneaking veggies into our kids' diet, we definitely like making the most out of snack time. Let's be honest—sometimes we would all rather eat our greens in cookie form.

6 tablespoons butter, softened

¼ cup brown sugar

1 egg

1 teaspoon vanilla extract

1 cup shredded zucchini

1 cup unbleached all-purpose flour

1 teaspoon baking powder

1 teaspoon cinnamon

¼ teaspoon salt

2 cups old-fashioned oats

1 cup mini chocolate chips

1. Preheat the oven to 350°F. Line two baking sheets with parchment paper.

2. In a large bowl using an electric mixer (or in a stand mixer using the paddle attachment), whip together the butter and sugar until light and fluffy, about 2 minutes. Add the egg and vanilla extract, and mix until combined. Stir in the zucchini.

3. In a medium bowl, add the flour, baking powder, cinnamon, and salt. Whisk to combine. Add the dry mixture to the zucchini mixture and stir to combine. Fold in the oats and chocolate chips.

4. Scoop the dough, about 2 tablespoons at a time, onto the prepared baking sheet, leaving a few inches between cookies.

5. Bake for 12 to 15 minutes, until lightly brown and set in the center. Cool before serving.

6. Store leftovers in a sealed container at room temperature for 2 days, or in the refrigerator for up to a week.

TIP: These cookies freeze well from the dough stage or after baking. To freeze cookie dough, scoop the dough onto the prepared pan, and freeze until dough is firm. Transfer frozen dough balls to a freezer-safe container and freeze up to 3 months. Bake from frozen according to directions, adding about 10 minutes to the baking time.

CRANBERRY PISTACHIO GRANOLA BARS

FREEZER-FRIENDLY, DAIRY-FREE, GLUTEN-FREE, VEGAN
YIELDS 1 (8-BY-8-INCH) PAN

Christmas in July? Why not! These beautiful red and green whole food granola bars are delicious any time of year, and the flavor combination of pistachios and cranberries is timeless.

1 cup old-fashioned oats	1 cup shelled pistachios	1 teaspoon vanilla extract
1 cup pitted dates	3 tablespoons coconut oil, plus more as needed	½ cup unsweetened dried cranberries, chopped

1. Line an 8-by-8-inch square pan with parchment paper.

2. In a food processor, combine the oats, dates, pistachios, coconut oil, and vanilla extract. Pulse until mixture is well combined and begins to stick together, until it forms a ball when squeezed. (If the mixture seems too crumbly and does not stick together, add coconut oil or water, 1 teaspoon at a time, until it does.)

3. Transfer to a large bowl and fold in the dried cranberries. Press into the prepared pan and refrigerate until firm. Slice into bars and serve.

4. Individually wrap granola bars in waxed paper and store in the refrigerator for up to 1 week or the freezer for up to 3 months. These can be taken on the go without refrigeration.

TIP: Make these ahead of time and wrap them in wax paper for a quick breakfast or snacks on a family trip, or drizzle them with melted white chocolate for a decadent dessert at home.

FROZEN YOGURT BARK

FREEZER-FRIENDLY, GLUTEN-FREE, NUT-FREE, VEGETARIAN
YIELDS 2 CUPS

A simple snack perfect for warm weather, frozen yogurt bark is one of our go-tos recipes. This recipe is extremely versatile, so substitute whatever fruit you have available. Try mixing in your favorite breakfast cereal or granola for an extra crunch.

1 cup plain or vanilla whole milk Greek yogurt

1 cup blueberries or chopped strawberries

1. Line a rimmed baking sheet with parchment paper.

2. In a medium bowl, combine the yogurt and fruit, and stir to combine.

3. Pour the fruit and yogurt mixture onto the prepared baking sheet, and spread into a thin layer with a spatula. Freeze until firm.

4. Serve directly from the freezer, breaking the bark into chunks.

5. Freeze leftover bark in a freezer-safe bag for up to 3 months.

CHOCOLATE CHIA PUDDING

DAIRY-FREE, NUT-FREE, GLUTEN-FREE, VEGAN
YIELDS 2 CUPS

If you haven't checked out chia pudding yet, we highly recommend it. Chia seeds are an awesome source of iron, fiber, and protein, and they thicken into a creamy, pudding-like texture when mixed with milk. We like using full-fat coconut milk for extra richness.

1½ cups full-fat coconut milk

2 tablespoons unsweetened cocoa powder

½ teaspoon vanilla extract

2 tablespoons maple syrup (optional)

½ cup chia seeds

1. In a large bowl with a tight-fitting lid, whisk together the coconut milk, cocoa powder, vanilla extract, and maple syrup (if using), until well combined. Add the chia seeds and whisk again until combined.

2. Cover and refrigerate overnight. Alternatively, pour into individual jars or containers with tight-fitting lids for single serving portions.

TIP: Swap out the maple syrup for a mashed ripe banana to enjoy naturally sweetened banana-flavored pudding.

CHOCOLATE CHIP BANANA BREAD

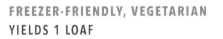

FREEZER-FRIENDLY, VEGETARIAN
YIELDS 1 LOAF

Is there anything more kid-friendly than banana bread? While BLW children tend to surprise bystanders with their adventurous eating skills, there is still plenty of room to serve classic kid favorites as well. This bread is decadently moist and flavorful, dotted with chocolate chips and finely chopped walnuts for added crunch.

1 cup mashed ripe banana (about 3 medium bananas)

½ cup butter, melted (1 stick)

¼ cup sugar

2 eggs

½ cup plain whole milk Greek yogurt

2 teaspoons vanilla extract

1½ cups unbleached all-purpose flour (or 1 cup all-purpose flour plus ½ cup whole-wheat flour)

1 teaspoon baking soda

¼ teaspoon salt

½ cup mini chocolate chips (optional)

½ cup walnuts, finely chopped (optional)

1. Preheat oven to 350°F. Line a loaf pan with parchment paper.

2. In a large bowl, stir together the mashed banana, butter, and sugar. Mix in the eggs, yogurt, and vanilla extract, and stir until well combined.

3. In a medium bowl, whisk together the flour, baking soda, and salt until well combined. Pour the dry ingredients into the banana mixture and stir until just combined.

4. Fold in the chocolate chips and walnuts (if using).

5. Scrape the batter into the prepared pan and bake for 50 to 60 minutes, or until a toothpick inserted in the center comes out clean.

6. Refrigerate leftovers in a container with a tightly fitting lid for up to 3 days. Or wrap loaf tightly with plastic wrap and store in a freezer-safe container for up to 3 months.

PIZZA HUMMUS

DAIRY-FREE, GLUTEN-FREE, NUT-FREE, VEGAN
YIELDS 4 CUPS

Blending all the traditional pizza spices into a creamy hummus dip makes for a delicious snack or side dish. Have a dipping party with your toddler, using thin strips of crisp bell peppers, sweet cucumbers, tangy olive halves, or soft pita strips.

1 tablespoon extra-virgin olive oil

¼ cup tomato paste

2 teaspoons dried oregano

1 teaspoon dried basil

2 or 3 garlic cloves, peeled

3 cups canned chickpeas, drained and rinsed, ½ cup liquid reserved

¼ cup tahini

¼ cup fresh lemon juice

Salt

1. In a small skillet over medium-high heat, heat the olive oil. Add the tomato paste, oregano, and basil and cook for about 2 minutes, so the flavors can blend.

2. Spoon the mixture into a food processor, and add the garlic, chickpeas and reserved liquid, tahini, lemon juice, and salt. Purée until smooth.

3. Refrigerate leftovers in a sealed container for up to 3 days.

TIP: Think portable pizza. Use it as a dip for broccoli, cucumbers, carrots, or naan bread. Or enjoy this unique spread on a sandwich.

ROASTED CHICKPEAS

DAIRY-FREE, GLUTEN-FREE, NUT-FREE, VEGAN
YIELDS 2½ CUPS CHICKPEAS

Roasted chickpeas are a great salty, crunchy snack for all ages. Chickpeas are packed with protein, fiber, and iron. They are also high in calories and carbohydrates, making them a great snack for little tums. Move over, Cheerios and cheese puffs—there's a new portable snack in town.

2 (15-ounce) cans chickpeas, drained and rinsed, or 2½ cups cooked dried chickpeas

1 to 2 tablespoons extra-virgin olive oil

1 teaspoon garlic powder

½ teaspoon cumin

½ teaspoon paprika

1. Preheat the oven to 400°F. Line a rimmed baking sheet with parchment paper.

2. In a bowl, toss the chickpeas with the olive oil, garlic powder, cumin, and paprika. Spread the chickpeas in a single layer on the prepared baking sheet.

3. Bake for 35 to 45 minutes or until dried and crunchy. Let cool before serving.

4. Refrigerate leftovers in a sealed container for up to 3 days.

TIP: For younger babies, use more oil and reduce roasting time for a seasoned chickpea that is nice and soft. For older toddlers, use less oil and roast longer for a light and crispy snack.

PARMESAN BAKED EDAMAME

GLUTEN-FREE, NUT-FREE, VEGETARIAN
YIELDS 2 CUPS EDAMAME

Edamame is simply the immature soybean. It's also a complete protein source filled with fiber, and it's a great on-the-go snack for young eaters. This recipe adds a warm, savory spin that still focuses on real food ingredients—a welcome replacement for the commonly promoted synthetic "vegetable crisp."

1 (12-ounce) package fresh or frozen shelled edamame

1 tablespoon extra-virgin olive oil

¼ cup grated Parmesan cheese

¼ teaspoon garlic powder

¼ teaspoon salt

¼ teaspoon freshly ground black pepper

1. Preheat the oven to 400°F. Line a rimmed baking sheet with parchment paper.

2. If using frozen edamame, thaw in refrigerator, rinse in a colander, and dry thoroughly on paper towels.

3. In a medium bowl, toss the edamame with the olive oil, cheese, garlic powder, salt, and pepper, mixing well.

4. Evenly spread the edamame on the prepared baking sheet. Bake for 25 to 30 minutes or until desired crispness. Serve immediately for best quality.

5. Refrigerate leftovers in a sealed container for up to 3 days. The edamame will soften in storage but can be reheated in the oven to reach desired crispness.

CREAMY CORN OFF THE COB

GLUTEN-FREE, NUT-FREE, VEGETARIAN
YIELDS 4 TO 6 CUPS

This recipe is an adaptation of traditional Mexican street corn, which is typically fire-roasted on the cob and then spread with crema (similar to sour cream), piquant Cotija cheese, and various spices. In our version, we use frozen corn for convenience and to make it baby-friendly. For a more authentic-tasting recipe, use fresh grilled corn; you can cut off the kernels or leave the cobs whole and coat them with the dressing and spices in the traditional manner!

2 tablespoons butter

1 tablespoon minced garlic

½ medium red onion, diced

2 or 3 (12-ounce) bags frozen corn

Salt

Freshly ground black pepper

2 tablespoons mayonnaise

2 tablespoons plain Greek yogurt

2 tablespoons lime juice

Cayenne pepper (optional)

Chili powder (optional)

4 ounces Cotija cheese, crumbled

Fresh cilantro, for garnish (optional)

1. In a cast-iron skillet over medium-high heat, melt the butter. Add the garlic, red onion, and frozen corn. Spread evenly in the skillet and flatten on top. Wait 2 to 3 minutes before stirring, allow vegetables to brown a little. Stir and repeat. Season with salt and pepper to taste.

2. In a small bowl, combine the mayonnaise, yogurt, lime juice, and cayenne pepper and powder (if using). Stir into the cooked corn. Sprinkle with Cotija cheese and garnish with cilantro (if using). Serve warm.

3. Refrigerate leftovers in a container with a tightly fitting lid for up to 2 days.

TIP: Substitute crema for the mayo and Greek yogurt if your grocer carries it. And if you can't find Cotija cheese, you can substitute grated Romano or crumbled feta.

CREAMY BAKED BRUSSELS SPROUTS

GLUTEN-FREE, NUT-FREE
YIELDS ABOUT 4 TO 6 CUPS

This recipe sheds a whole new light on this humble veggie. They are like no Brussels sprouts you've ever tasted. We think they'll convert the most anti-sprout people into believers, and your toddler won't have any reason to become a critic. But don't take our word for it. Try it for yourself!

4 bacon slices, cooked crisp and roughly chopped, drippings reserved

½ medium onion, finely diced

½ teaspoon minced garlic

1½ pounds Brussels sprouts, halved, stems cut off

½ teaspoon salt

½ teaspoon freshly ground black pepper

½ cup heavy cream

6 ounces sharp white Cheddar cheese, grated

1. Preheat the oven to 375°F.

2. In a cast-iron skillet over medium heat, add the bacon drippings. Add the onion and garlic and sauté for about 4 minutes, stirring frequently, until translucent and tender.

3. Add the Brussels sprouts and cook until bright green and slightly tender, 8 to 10 minutes. Sprinkle with salt and pepper.

4. Remove the skillet from heat, pour the heavy cream over the sprouts, then top with cheese and chopped bacon.

5. Bake for 15 to 17 minutes, until the cheese is bubbly and Brussels sprouts are as tender as you desire. Serve warm.

6. Refrigerate leftovers in a sealed container for up to 3 days.

TIP: This recipe is also delicious when Brussels sprouts are substituted with any cruciferous vegetable, like cauliflower or broccoli.

BUTTERNUT SQUASH RISOTTO

FREEZER-FRIENDLY, GLUTEN-FREE, NUT-FREE
YIELDS 8 CUPS

Butternut squash is beautifully rich in nutrition and flavor, and this recipe is likely to become a family favorite. The squash has a naturally melt-in-your-mouth texture that makes it a star ingredient in many BLW-friendly recipes and as a stand-alone side dish, and is just one of the many reasons it remains a staple in our kitchens.

1 medium butternut squash

2 tablespoons extra-virgin olive oil

½ teaspoon salt, plus more to taste

Freshly ground black pepper, divided

8 cups low-sodium vegetable broth, divided

3 tablespoons butter

1 medium onion, diced

1½ cups Arborio rice

⅛ teaspoon turmeric

¼ cup heavy cream

½ cup grated or shaved Parmesan cheese, plus more for garnish

Minced parsley, for garnish

1. Preheat the oven to 400°F. Line a rimmed baking sheet with parchment paper.

2. Carefully cut the squash in half lengthwise. Scoop out seeds with a spoon or ice cream scoop. Gently score the squash with a knife, drizzle with olive oil, and season with the salt and pepper. Place the squash on the prepared baking sheet and roast for 45 to 60 minutes, until it is fork-tender in the thickest part of the squash. Let cool 30 to 45 minutes.

3. Scoop the cooled squash flesh from the skin into a large bowl. Use a hand-held mixer to blend the squash with 2 cups of vegetable broth until smooth. Set aside.

4. In a medium pot over low heat, or in a glass bowl in a microwave, heat the remaining vegetable broth. Keep warm.

5. In a large pot over medium heat, melt the butter. Add the onions and cook until translucent, 2 to 3 minutes. Add the Arborio rice and stir, cooking for 1 minute. Reduce heat to low. In 1-cup increments, add the remaining vegetable broth to the skillet, stirring continuously while the broth is slowly absorbed. Continue until all 6 cups have been added and the rice starts to become tender. Season with salt and pepper and taste for desired tenderness.

6. When the rice is done, gently stir in the semi-pureed squash and season with the turmeric. Pour in the heavy cream and add the cheese, stirring until just combined. Taste and add more salt and pepper as needed. Sprinkle parsley over the top and serve immediately.

7. Store in a sealed container in the refrigerator for 5 to 7 days. Freeze in an airtight container for up to 3 months.

TIP: This recipe's mild flavor makes it perfect as a complementary side dish at supper or a savory addition to breakfast.

BUTTERNUT SQUASH SOUP

GLUTEN-FREE, NUT-FREE
YIELDS 6 CUPS

Soup is a great option to include in your baby's meals; it's tasty and can be so packed with nutrients, especially when made with fiber-filled squash. This one is creamy and delicious. See the Tip for ideas on serving soup to babies.

6 tablespoons butter or coconut oil

1 onion, diced

1 garlic clove, minced

1 large (2- to 2½-pound) butternut squash, skin removed, seeded, and cut into cubes

4 cups low-sodium vegetable or chicken broth

½ teaspoon ground nutmeg

½ teaspoon freshly ground black pepper

½ cup heavy cream

1. In a Dutch oven over medium heat, melt the butter. Add the onion and garlic and cook, stirring frequently, until fragrant, about 3 minutes.

2. Add the butternut squash, broth, nutmeg, and pepper. Cover and simmer until squash is tender, about 15 minutes.

3. With an immersion blender, blend soup until smooth. Stir in the heavy cream. Serve warm.

4. To store, refrigerate in a sealed container for up to 3 days, or in individual portions that you can reheat for quick lunches.

TIP: Here are a few ideas for offering soup during baby-led weaning:
- Serve as a topping or dip for strips or slices of bread.
- Offer in preloaded spoons.
- Add in a can of rinsed and drained chickpeas and blend. This makes creamy soups much thicker and easier to scoop.

BAKED POTATO SOUP

NUT-FREE
YIELDS 12 TO 14 CUPS

A thick and creamy baked potato soup is a great starter soup for little ones. Its rich consistency will cling to the spoon, and it has a mild flavor for any palate. Soups are great during bouts of teething because they usually require minimal chewing but still provide what's needed for quality energy.

4 large potatoes

⅔ cup butter

⅔ cup all-purpose flour

7 cups milk

4 scallions, chopped, reserving some for garnish

12 slices bacon, cooked and crumbled, reserving some for garnish

1¼ cups shredded Cheddar cheese, reserving some for garnish

1 cup plain Greek yogurt

1 teaspoon salt

1 teaspoon freshly ground black pepper

1. Preheat the oven to 400°F.

2. Wrap the potatoes in aluminum foil and bake for 45 to 55 minutes. Let cool, then cube. Set aside.

3. In a large stockpot, melt the butter over medium heat. Whisk in the flour until smooth. Slowly stir in the milk, whisking constantly until thick.

4. In a medium bowl, roughly mash half of the cubed potatoes, and stir them into the milk mixture, along with the remaining potatoes and scallions. Bring to a boil, stirring frequently. Reduce heat to medium-low, cover, and simmer for about 10 minutes.

5. Fold in the bacon, cheese, yogurt, salt, and pepper, stirring frequently, until cheese is melted.

6. Garnish with reserved bacon, scallions, and cheese before serving. Refrigerate leftovers in a sealed container for up to 3 days.

TWICE-BAKED SAVORY SWEET POTATOES

NUT-FREE, VEGETARIAN
YIELDS 4 POTATO HALVES

Another sweet potato recipe? Yes, indeed. It's worth including because it's OH. SO. GOOD. The savory spin on a traditionally sweet dish makes this recipe unique. The vibrant orange and green scream beta-carotene and iron, two key players for lifelong nutrition. Also, this dish is multi-textural, with its creamy sweet potato flesh, crunchy potato skins, tender cooked greens, and chewy chickpeas.

2 large sweet potatoes
1½ tablespoons butter
½ medium onion, finely chopped
2 cups fresh baby spinach

2 ounces cream cheese
¼ cup whole milk Greek yogurt
1 cup canned chickpeas, rinsed and drained
¼ teaspoon salt

¼ teaspoon freshly ground black pepper
Extra-virgin olive oil, for coating the skins
¼ cup shredded mozzarella cheese

1. Preheat the oven to 350°F.

2. Wrap the sweet potatoes in aluminum foil and bake for 45 to 60 minutes. Once baked, let them cool for 5 to 10 minutes.

3. While sweet potatoes are cooling, melt the butter and sauté the onion over medium heat until translucent. Add the spinach and cook for 2 to 3 minutes, stirring continuously, until tender. Set aside.

4. Remove the foil from the sweet potatoes and cut them in half lengthwise. Scrape the sweet potato flesh into a mixing bowl, leaving a thin layer of flesh inside the peel so it can stand up on its own.

5. Using a handheld mixer, whip the sweet potato flesh with the cream cheese and yogurt. Stir in the chickpeas, spinach and onion mixture, salt, and pepper.

6. Coat the outside of the potato skins with a drizzle of olive oil and bake for 5 to 10 minutes to crisp. Remove from oven and fill each skin with the sweet potato mixture. Top with the mozzarella cheese. Bake again for 10 to 15 minutes, or until cheese is melted and filling is heated through. Serve warm.

7. Refrigerate leftovers in a container with a tightly fitting lid for up to 3 days.

TIP: If you have room in your fridge, you can semi-prep these ahead of time by storing the empty sweet potato skins and filling separately. On serving day, throw the skins into the oven and bake until crispy. Stuff the skins with the creamy filling, top with mozzarella, and bake again.

BETTER-THAN-BOXED MACARONI AND CHEESE

NUT-FREE, VEGETARIAN
YIELDS 4 CUPS

While we definitely don't mind boxed mac and cheese from time to time, we were surprised by how simple this family favorite is to make at home. We hope this recipe will be your go-to for a quick version of this favorite pasta dish.

8 ounces elbow macaroni noodles, or other small pasta

¼ cup butter

¼ cup unbleached all-purpose flour

2 cups milk

2 cups shredded Cheddar cheese

1. Cook pasta according to package directions. Drain and set aside.

2. In a large saucepan over medium heat, melt the butter. Stir in the flour and whisk constantly until the mixture is smooth and lightly golden brown, about 5 minutes.

3. Slowly add the milk to the flour mixture, stirring continuously, until mixture is smooth and thickened, about 5 minutes.

4. Add the cheese and stir until melted, 2 to 4 minutes.

5. Add the pasta to the cheese sauce and stir to coat. Serve warm.

6. Store leftovers in a sealed container in the refrigerator for up to 3 days.

NOTE: Change up this recipe by using a different combination of cheeses such as Monterey Jack or mozzarella. To make a veggie-loaded version, add finely chopped broccoli florets, finely chopped fresh or frozen spinach, or a handful of frozen peas to the boiling pasta 1 to 2 minutes before straining.

TEXAS CAVIAR

DAIRY-FREE, GLUTEN-FREE, NUT-FREE, VEGETARIAN
YIELDS ABOUT 10 CUPS

Here it is: your family's newest summertime staple. Every picnic, cookout, barbecue, potluck, or birthday party—you name it, just make it. Although the prep time involves a fair amount of chopping, the outcome is marvelous. Invest in a sharp chef's knife, turn on some Beach Boys songs, and you're set. Fresh, crisp veggies, fiber-filled beans, and tangy vinegar dressing—it's a party in a bowl the whole family will enjoy, right down to your little one.

For the dressing

½ cup granulated sugar

¾ cup apple cider vinegar

1 teaspoon water

½ cup extra-virgin olive oil

For the salad

1½ cups fresh corn kernels (cut from 2 large ears)

1 cup very finely chopped celery (4 or 5 stalks)

1 cup diced green pepper

1 cup diced red, orange, or yellow bell pepper

¾ cup diced red onion

1 (15-ounce) can pinto beans

1 (15-ounce) can black beans

1 (15-ounce) can chickpeas

1 (15-ounce) can black-eyed peas

2 (4-ounce) cans mild chopped green chiles

Salt (optional)

Freshly ground black pepper

To make the dressing

1. Combine the dressing ingredients in a saucepan and bring to a boil, stirring occasionally.

2. Let boil for 1 to 2 minutes, remove heat, and let cool to room temperature. It will smell strongly of vinegar, but do not add more sugar.

To make the salad

3. Add all the salad ingredients to a large bowl with a tightly fitting lid, and mix well. Top with the vinaigrette and stir again until well combined. Refrigerate for at least one hour, or ideally overnight.

4. Serve the salad by itself or with whole-grain tortilla chips as an appetizer or quick snack.

5. This salad can be stored in the refrigerator for up to 3 days.

RED BEANS AND RICE

FREEZER-FRIENDLY, GLUTEN-FREE, NUT-FREE
YIELDS ABOUT 20 CUPS

A personal note from Ellen: "This recipe has been a family favorite for over 30 years. The basis of it was given to my father by a Cajun chef he met on an airplane flying back to New Orleans. It has been modified slightly through the years, getting better with each innovation. Most who have tried it agree to its supremacy. Well representing all the major food groups, it's almost a complete meal in itself, but definitely benefits from some pan-fried cornbread and butter on the side. We make this recipe mild, knowing that the diner can add as much heat as they wish. There was a period in my family's history where we made this every Tuesday night before a weekly mission trip to Cairo, Illinois." (Note that while traditional red beans and rice typically has sausages cut into thin coins, this method isn't baby-friendly. Make sure you cut them into smaller pieces!)

5 cups water
1 tablespoon butter
2½ cups brown rice
4 (15-ounce) cans dark red kidney beans
1 (15-ounce) can light red kidney beans
1 pound smoked kielbasa beef sausage, cut lengthwise into quarters and sliced crosswise

2 large onions, diced
5 stalks celery, thinly sliced
1 jalapeño or 8 slices jalapeño, diced
2 garlic cloves, peeled, or 1 teaspoon minced garlic
2 tablespoons liquid smoke
5 tablespoon ketchup
1 tablespoon cumin

1 teaspoon freshly ground black pepper
½ teaspoon cayenne pepper
½ teaspoon dried basil
½ teaspoon dried thyme
½ teaspoon dried parsley
½ teaspoon fresh rosemary, chopped

1. Bring the water to a boil, and add the butter. Stir in the brown rice, reduce heat to low, cover, and let simmer for 30 minutes. When water is almost evaporated, turn off heat and let steam until ready to serve.

2. In a large Dutch oven or slow cooker, add all the remaining ingredients, and bring to a low boil. Let juices cook down, and stir continuously for 60 to 90 minutes.

3. Serve the bean mixture atop warm brown rice.

4. Store leftovers in a sealed container in the refrigerator for up to 3 days. Freeze in individual containers for up to 3 months.

TIP: Garnish this dish with scallions and serve with sweet green peas. You can also substitute Cajun-style andouille sausage for the kielbasa.

CAROLYN'S WHITE CHILI

GLUTEN-FREE, NUT-FREE
YIELDS 12 TO 14 CUPS

A not-so-classic white chicken chili is one of the best fall foods. This recipe tastes best when made by a grandma (trust us), so it's definitely one to share with the whole family. Serve with a crisp green salad of cranberries and apples, along with a hearty chunk of French bread (once your baby has some teeth) for lots of sopping, and you're set!

1 tablespoon extra-virgin olive oil

2 medium onions, diced

2 (4-ounce) cans mild chopped green chiles

4 garlic cloves, minced

1½ tablespoons dried oregano, crumbled

2 teaspoons cumin

¼ teaspoon cayenne pepper

3 (16-ounce) cans great northern beans, undrained

6 cups low-sodium chicken broth

4 cups shredded cooked chicken

3 cups grated Monterey Jack cheese (approximately 12 ounces)

Salt

Freshly ground black pepper

Sour cream or plain Greek yogurt for garnish

1. In a large stockpot over medium-high heat, heat the oil. Add the onions and sauté until translucent, 7 to 8 minutes. Stir in the chiles, garlic, oregano, cumin, and cayenne pepper, and sauté an additional 2 minutes.

2. Add the beans and chicken broth, and bring to a boil. Reduce heat, add the chicken and cheese, and stir continuously until cheese is melted. Season with salt and pepper.

3. Garnish with sour cream or Greek yogurt when serving.

TIP: Using a rotisserie chicken and canned beans makes this a semi-quick dish, but with soup and chili, the longer the flavors can simmer and marinate, the better, so this recipe also works great in a slow cooker.

PAPPY'S CHILI

NUT-FREE
YIELDS 12 TO 14 CUPS

This is a treasured dish from Ellen's family. This recipe, attributed to her reigning patriarch, Pappy, actually originates from his mother. Never satisfied to leave well enough alone, Pappy perpetually experimented and fine-tuned his mother's gift until he found what he thought to be the best rendition thereof. We hope you agree and continue the journey—feel free to make this recipe your own.

For the seasoning

2 tablespoons plus 1 teaspoon chili powder

1 tablespoon plus 1 teaspoon ground cumin

2 teaspoons salt

1 teaspoon onion powder

½ teaspoon cayenne pepper

½ teaspoon garlic powder

½ teaspoon freshly ground black pepper

For the chili

2 pounds ground beef

Homemade chili seasoning or 2 (1.25-ounce) packages chili seasoning

1 medium onion, diced

½ teaspoon minced garlic

3 (15-ounce) cans chili beans, undrained

1 (15-ounce) can red kidney beans, undrained

2 (16-ounce) cans tomato sauce

Salt

Freshly ground black pepper

1 (10-ounce) can diced tomato and green chile blend

½ pound uncooked dry spaghetti noodles, broken into thirds (optional)

To make the seasoning

In a small bowl, mix together all the ingredients and set aside.

To make the chili

1. In a large cast-iron Dutch oven, brown the meat, using a spoon to make the smallest bits possible. Drain excess grease.

2. Add the chili seasoning to the meat. Add the onion and garlic and stir until lightly brown.

3. Add the beans and tomato sauce, and simmer on low. Add salt and pepper to taste.

4. Add the tomatoes and continue to simmer for 45 to 60 minutes, stirring frequently.

5. Stir in the dry spaghetti noodles, bring to a boil, and boil until al dente, stirring very frequently or food will scorch. As you stir, taste test. When it tastes thick and rich, remove from heat. Serve warm.

6. Refrigerate leftovers in a sealed container for up to 3 days, or freeze in individual containers for up to 3 months.

TIP: You can also make this chili in a slow cooker, where you will not need to stir it as much. The variations for this dish are endless. Garnish with plain Greek yogurt, shredded Cheddar cheese, and extra hot sauce, and serve with hot corn bread pancakes (just mix up a box of Jiffy corn bread and pour onto a hot greased griddle). This is a thick chili recipe, so the longer you can cook the juices down, the better. And, for a fun Cincinnati-style chili twist (this is where the spaghetti addition comes from), throw in a pinch of cinnamon with the other spices.

MEXICAN CHICKEN CASSEROLE

FREEZER-FRIENDLY, NUT-FREE
YIELDS 1 (9-BY-13-INCH) CASSEROLE

The best recipes you'll ever discover are hidden within the pages of church or community cookbooks. Ellen's family has been making this chicken casserole for over 30 years. No fancy, trendy ingredients, just a tried-and-true tasty recipe. It makes a great family weeknight meal served with a side of our Basic Black Beans (page 76) and So-Good Guacamole (page 70).

2 (10.5-ounce) cans cream of chicken soup

1 (10-ounce) can diced tomato and green chile blend, divided

1 teaspoon salt

1 teaspoon freshly ground black pepper

1 tablespoon butter

1 large onion, diced

1 tablespoon minced garlic

1 cup chicken broth

8 ounces button mushrooms, roughly chopped

1½ pounds tender cooked chicken, diced small or shredded, divided

2½ cups shredded Cheddar cheese, divided

1. Heat the soup. Add the tomatoes, salt, pepper, and chicken broth. Boil on low for 5 to 7 minutes, until slightly thickened.

2. In a small skillet over medium-high heat, melt the butter. Add the onions, garlic, and mushrooms and cook until tender, about 5 minutes. Divide onion/mushroom mixture for the next step.

3. Preheat the oven to 375°F. In a greased 9-by-13-inch casserole dish, layer with half each of the chicken, the onion/mushroom mixture, cheese, and tomatoes. Repeat with the remaining ingredients.

4. Bake for about 30 minutes, until cheese and sauce are bubbly. Serve warm.

5. Refrigerate leftovers for up to 3 days, or cool and wrap tightly in plastic wrap and freeze for up to 3 months.

SALMON PASTA WITH PEANUT SAUCE

DAIRY-FREE

YIELDS 6 TO 8 CUPS

Although it's toddler-friendly, this dish doubles as a date-night quality dinner made at home. This everyday gourmet recipe takes several staple cupboard ingredients and gives mealtime a new fantastic point of view. This peanut sauce will open you up to a whole new world of potential pasta sauces.

For the peanut sauce

1 cup full-fat coconut milk

⅓ cup creamy peanut butter

3 tablespoons brown sugar

1 tablespoon reduced-sodium soy sauce

1 tablespoon apple cider vinegar

1 teaspoon garlic powder

½ teaspoon ground ginger

For the pasta and salmon

16 ounces whole-wheat spaghetti or other long pasta

1 teaspoon sesame oil

1 medium red bell pepper, sliced into strips

4 teaspoons minced garlic

1 pound boneless, skinless salmon fillets, cut into 1-inch chunks

4 teaspoons peeled, minced fresh ginger or ¼ teaspoon ground ginger

½ teaspoon salt

½ teaspoon freshly ground black pepper

2 cups chopped kale or other dark greens

3 tablespoons finely chopped cilantro (optional)

To make the peanut sauce

In a medium bowl, whisk together the peanut sauce ingredients until thoroughly blended. Set aside.

To make the pasta and salmon

1. Cook pasta according to package directions; drain.

2. In a large nonstick skillet over medium-high heat, briefly heat the oil. Add the bell pepper and garlic, and sauté for 3 to 4 minutes. Add the salmon, ginger, salt, and pepper, and cook for about 2 minutes, stirring occasionally. Stir in the kale.

3. Add the peanut sauce and cook for about 3 minutes more, stirring occasionally, until the salmon is cooked through, tender, and flaky, and the sauce has thickened slightly.

4. Serve the salmon mixture over pasta and sprinkled with cilantro (if using).

5. Refrigerate leftovers in a container with a tightly fitting lid for up to 3 days.

TIP: You can mix the peanut sauce up to a day ahead and store it, covered, in the refrigerator. You can also pre-chop the veggies for a super-quick supper.

CRUNCHY COCONUT FISH STICKS

DAIRY-FREE, NUT-FREE
YIELDS 16 STRIPS

Laura's memories of fish sticks come from sleepovers at her grandma's house, where tidy little sticks came from a yellow bag in the freezer. This recipe is a homemade variation that allows you to control the ingredients—in this case, with delicious coconut.

½ cup panko breadcrumbs

½ cup unsweetened shredded coconut

½ teaspoon garlic powder

½ teaspoon onion powder

½ teaspoon freshly ground black pepper

1 egg

1 pound tilapia or halibut, sliced into sticks

2 to 3 tablespoons extra-virgin olive oil

1. Preheat the oven to 350°F. Line a rimmed baking sheet with parchment paper.

2. In a shallow container, such as a pie pan, combine the breadcrumbs, coconut, garlic powder, onion powder, and pepper, and stir until mixed.

3. In a small bowl, whisk the egg until lightly beaten.

4. Dip the fish sticks into the egg, and then roll in the coconut and breadcrumb mixture until well coated. Place breaded fish sticks on the prepared baking sheet and drizzle with olive oil.

5. Bake for 10 to 12 minutes or until lightly browned. Serve warm.

6. Store leftovers in a tightly sealed container in the refrigerator for 2 to 3 days.

STICK-TO-YOUR-RIBS BEEF STEW

DAIRY-FREE, NUT-FREE

YIELDS 12 TO 14 CUPS

This homemade beef stew is hearty, flavorful, and most likely tastes unlike any you've had before. Another one of Ellen's family-favorite one-pot wonders, this recipe will keep all the kiddos happy and satisfied well after supper. Although it's a time investment, it really is worth it, and the leftovers taste even better!

2 pounds lean beef chuck, trimmed and cut into 1-inch strips

2 tablespoons all-purpose flour

1 tablespoon extra-virgin olive oil, plus more if needed

2 large onions, sliced into rings (about 3 cups)

2 garlic cloves, minced

1 tablespoon tomato paste

2 cups low-sodium beef broth

1 tablespoon dried parsley

½ teaspoon dried rosemary

½ teaspoon dried thyme

1 teaspoon salt

1 teaspoon freshly ground black pepper

4 cups diced carrots

4 or 5 russet potatoes, unpeeled, sliced into large circles

4 or 5 celery stalks, finely chopped

1½ cups green beans

1½ cups corn

1 tablespoon cold water

1 tablespoon cornstarch

1. Coat the beef with the flour, shaking off any excess. In a large, nonstick pot over medium-high heat, heat the oil. Add the beef and sauté until browned, about 6 minutes. Remove the beef from the pot.

2. Add the onions to the pot along with more olive oil (if needed), and sauté for 6 minutes. Add the garlic and stir for 1 minute.

3. Return the beef to the pot. Stir in the tomato paste, then the beef broth. Add enough water to just cover; bring to a boil.

4. Add the parsley, rosemary, thyme, salt, and pepper. Reduce heat to low and simmer until the beef is tender, about 30 minutes.

5. Add the carrots, potatoes, and celery. Cover partially and simmer for about an hour. Add the green beans and corn, and simmer for 15 minutes more.

6. In a small bowl, whisk the cold water and cornstarch into a slurry, being careful not to leave any lumps. Stir into the stew. Increase heat to medium-high and boil for about 5 minutes. Serve warm.

7. Refrigerate leftovers in a sealed container for up to 3 days.

TIP: This stew works with any vegetable. Clean out the kitchen and feel free to throw in any other veggies you find—fresh, frozen, or canned.

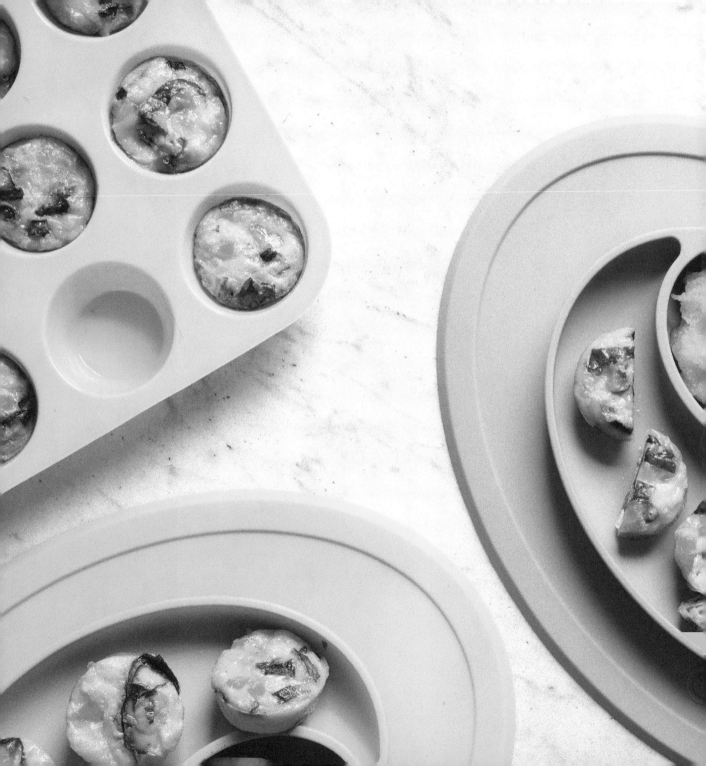

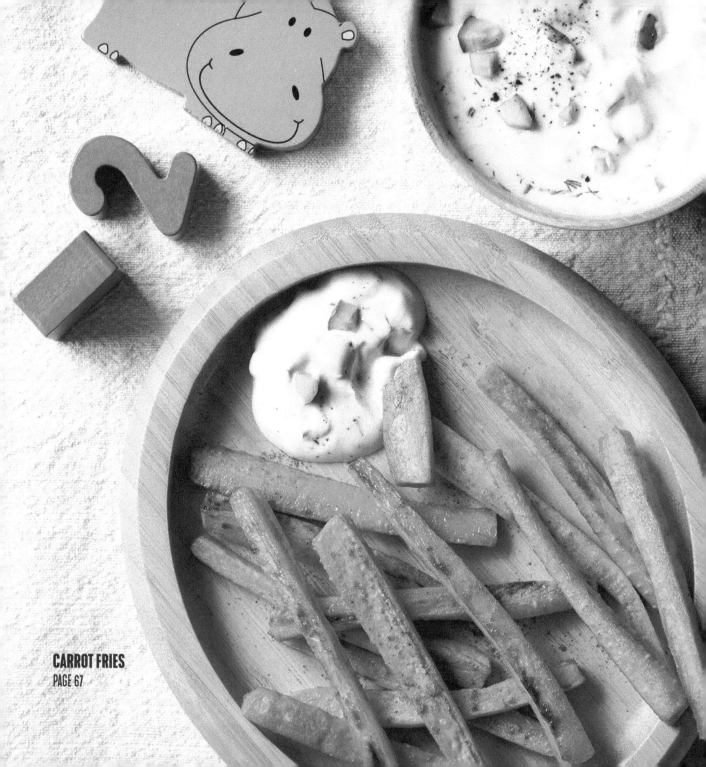

CARROT FRIES
PAGE 67

Measurement Conversions

VOLUME EQUIVALENTS (LIQUID)

US Standard	US Standard (ounces)	Metric (approximate)
2 tablespoons	1 fl. oz.	30 mL
¼ cup	2 fl. oz.	60 mL
½ cup	4 fl. oz.	120 mL
1 cup	8 fl. oz.	240 mL
1½ cups	12 fl. oz.	355 mL
2 cups or 1 pint	16 fl. oz.	475 mL
4 cups or 1 quart	32 fl. oz.	1 L
1 gallon	128 fl. oz.	4 L

OVEN TEMPERATURES

Fahrenheit	Celsius (approximate)
250°F	120°C
300°F	150°C
325°F	165°C
350°F	180°C
375°F	190°C
400°F	200°C
425°F	220°C
450°F	230°C

VOLUME EQUIVALENTS (DRY)

US Standard	Metric (approximate)
⅛ teaspoon	0.5 mL
¼ teaspoon	1 mL
½ teaspoon	2 mL
¾ teaspoon	4 mL
1 teaspoon	5 mL
1 tablespoon	15 mL
¼ cup	59 mL
⅓ cup	79 mL
½ cup	118 mL
⅔ cup	156 mL
¾ cup	177 mL
1 cup	235 mL
2 cups or 1 pint	475 mL
3 cups	700 mL
4 cups or 1 quart	1 L

WEIGHT EQUIVALENTS

US Standard	Metric (approximate)
½ ounce	15 g
1 ounce	30 g
2 ounces	60 g
4 ounces	115 g
8 ounces	225 g
12 ounces	340 g
16 ounces or 1 pound	455 g

Resources

Feeding Littles—A team of feeding experts (registered dietitian and occupational therapist) who offer baby-led weaning guidance on topics from motor development to constipation. www.feedinglittles.com

New Ways Nutrition—If you find you have a question or two that pop up during your baby-led weaning journey, there is a good chance Renae of New Ways Nutrition has a blog post about it. www.newwaysnutrition.com

Plant Based Juniors—If you are vegetarian, vegan, or predominantly plant-based, we recommend checking out this duo of dietitians who provide expert advice on meeting all of your plant-based baby's nutrient needs. www.plantbasedjuniors.com

Ellyn Satter Institute—Straightforward, easy-to-follow feeding advice from the registered dietitian and family therapist who created the gold standard in feeding children: the Division of Responsibility. www.ellynsatterinstitute.org

The Nourished Child—Jill Castle is a well-respected pediatric registered dietitian specializing in infant to teen nutrition. www.jillcastle.com/blog

The National Association of the Deaf— This organization encourages everyone to experience learning and using American Sign Language (ASL) and believes it is beneficial to people of all ages. www.nad.org/resources/american-sign-language

References

Academy of Nutrition and Dietetics. "Do's and Don'ts." *Eat Right*. December 2017. https://www.eatright.org/food/nutrition/eating-as-a-family/dos-and-donts-for-babys-first-foods.

American Academy of Allergy, Asthma & Immunology. "Food Intolerance versus Food Allergy." Accessed July 21, 2019. https://www.aaaai.org/conditions-and-treatments/library/allergy-library/food-intolerance.

American Academy of Pediatrics. "Breastfeeding and the Use of Human Milk." *Pediatrics* 129, no. 3 (March 2012). https://pediatrics.aappublications.org/content/129/3/e827.

American Academy of Pediatrics. "Starting Solid Foods." *Healthy Children*. Accessed July 21, 2019. https://www.healthychildren.org/English/ages-stages/baby/feeding-nutrition/Pages/Starting-Solid-Foods.aspx.

Anderson, Jane, and Den Trumbull. "The Benefits of the Family Table." Accessed July 21, 2019. https://www.acpeds.org/the-college-speaks/position-statements/parenting-issues/the-benefits-of-the-family-table.

Barrera, C. M., et al. "Timing of Introduction of Complementary Foods to US Infants, National Health and Nutrition Examination Survey 2009-2014." *Journal of the Academy of Nutrition and Dietetics* 118, no. 3 (March 2018): 464-70. doi: 10.1016/j.jand.2017.10.020.

Bennett, W. E., et al. "Early Cow's Milk Introduction Is Associated with Failed Personal-Social Milestones After One Year of Age." *European Journal of Pediatrics*. July 2014. https://doi.org/10.1007/s00431-014-2265-y.

Bravi, Francesca, et al. "Impact of maternal nutrition on breast-milk composition: A systematic review." *The American Journal of Clinical Nutrition* 104, no. 3 (September 2016). https://doi.org/10.3945/ajcn.115.120881.

Brown, A., and M. Lee. "Maternal child-feeding style during the weaning period: association with infant weight and maternal eating style." *Eating Behaviors*. April 2011. https://www.ncbi.nlm.nih.gov/pubmed/21385639.

Brown, Amy, Sarah Wyn Jones, and Hannah Rowan. "Baby-Led Weaning: The Evidence to Date." *Current Nutrition Reports*. April 29, 2017. https://www.ncbi.nlm.nih.gov/pmc/articles/PMC5438437.

Fangupo, Louise J., et al. "A Baby-Led Approach to Eating Solids and Risk of Choking." *Pediatrics* 138, no. 4 (October 2016). https://pediatrics.aappublications.org/content/pediatrics/138/4/e20160772.full.pdf.

Gupta, Ruchi S., et al. "The Public Health Impact of Parent-Reported Childhood Food Allergies in the United States." *Pediatrics* 142, no. 6 (December 2018). https://pediatrics.aappublications.org/content/142/6/e20181235.full.

Moorcroft, Kate, Joyce Marshall, and Felicia McCormick. "Association between timing of introducing solid foods and obesity in infancy and childhood: A systematic review." *Maternal & Child Nutrition* 7 (December 2010): 3-26. https://onlinelibrary.wiley.com/doi/full/10.1111/j.1740-8709.2010.00284.x.

Sicherer, Scott H., and Frank R. Greer. "Dietary interventions to prevent atopic disease: Updated recommendations." *AAP News*. March 18, 2019. https://www.aappublications.org/news/2019/03/18/atopy031819.

Sleep.org. "'Top Off' with Milk or Formula to Help Your Baby Sleep?" Accessed July 21, 2019. https://www.sleep.org/articles/top-off-with-milk-or-formula-to-help-your-baby-sleep/.

Townsend, Ellen, and Nicola J. Pitchford. "Baby knows best? The impact of weaning style on food preferences and body mass index in early childhood in a case-controlled sample." *BMJ Open* 2, no. 1 (January 2012). https://www.ncbi.nlm.nih.gov/pmc/articles/PMC4400680.

United States Department of Agriculture. "Organic Production & Handling Standards." USDA.gov. November 2016. https://www.ams.usda.gov/publications/content/organic-production-handling-standards.

Williams, Erickson L., et al. "Impact of a Modified Version of Baby-Led Weaning on Infant Food and Nutrient Intakes: The BLISS Randomized Controlled Trial." *Nutrients* 10, no. 6 (August 2018). https://www.mdpi.com/2072-6643/10/6/740/htm.

Index

Acknowledgments

FROM ELLEN

As the youngest child of four, I am 100 percent confident that this book never would have been possible without constant reinforcement, encouragement, supervision, and support from my family. To my dad, the most faithful book editor. To my husband, for always being the ping-pong paddle to my thoughts. To Ruthie, my busy, busy buzzing bee. You inspire me every day. To my sisters, for always taking care of me, no matter the age. To Laura, my co-author and "Ruthie mom" twin. Thank you for saying yes to this crazy project! To our readers, I am honored to share this message of health and opportunity and so many of my secret family recipes! To everyone in my life, I am grateful.

FROM LAURA

Thank you to my husband for helping me accomplish this crazy goal. To Ruthie and Bobby, my adventurous eaters. To all the dietitians out there for paving the way for us while sharing nutrition advice that's as reliable as it is awesome. And to my great friend and co-author, Ellen, for being so generous in sharing this opportunity.

About the Authors

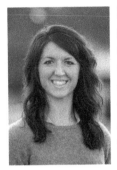

Ellen Gipson, MA, RDN, LD, is a registered dietitian, mom, and group fitness instructor. Beginning her dietetics career in school nutrition, Ellen championed the philosophy that food isn't nutritious unless eaten and early (and continual) exposure is essential in establishing healthy eating habits. After watching the pure joy on the face of her 8-month-old daughter chowing down on corn on the cob, she was inspired to lead other new parents and babies in their food adventures, founding her own company, Square One Wellness, and teaching local baby-led weaning workshops and classes. She lives in Cape Girardeau, Missouri, with her husband, Steve, daughter, Ruth, and the most prideful cat, Mr. Darcy.

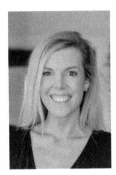

Laura Morton, MS, RDN, LD, is a registered dietitian and mom of two toddlers, both adventurous eaters. She shares her journey to peaceful mealtimes and positive food relationships through her blog and business, Morton's Grove. Like in other areas of parenting, Laura believes the goal of feeding is to cultivate a healthy relationship with food that lasts a lifetime. She shares this approach when counseling families with babies and toddlers. Laura and her family live in a 100-year-old farmhouse way out in the country, where you will almost always find them running around barefoot.